YOGA AND MINDFULNESS FOR YOUNG CHILDREN

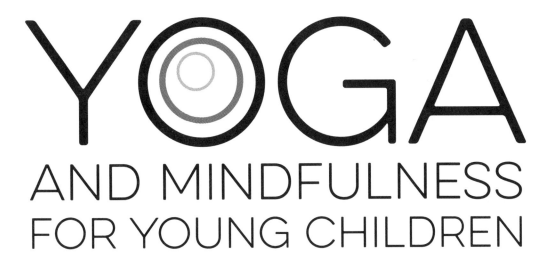

YOGA
AND MINDFULNESS
FOR YOUNG CHILDREN

Poses for Play,
Learning, and Peace

Maureen Heil and Ilene S. Rosen

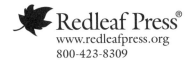 Redleaf Press®
www.redleafpress.org
800-423-8309

Published by Redleaf Press
10 Yorkton Court
St. Paul, MN 55117
www.redleafpress.org

First edition 2019
Senior editor: Heidi Hogg
Managing editor: Douglas Schmitz
Art director: Renee Hammes
Cover design: Louise OFarrell
Cover photograph: yaruta/Canva
Interior design: Michelle Lee Lagerroos
Typeset in Museo Slab and Museo Sans
Interior photos: Ilene S. Rosen

Printed in the United States of America
26 25 24 23 22 21 20 19   1 2 3 4 5 6 7 8

Library of Congress Cataloging-in-Publication Data

Names: Heil, Maureen, author. | Rosen, Ilene S., author.
Title: Yoga and mindfulness for young children : poses for play, learning, and peace / by Maureen Heil and Ilene S. Rosen.
Description: First edition. | St. Paul, MN : Redleaf Press, [2019] | Includes bibliographical references and index.
Identifiers: LCCN 2019013324 | ISBN 9781605546674 (pbk. : alk. paper)
Subjects: LCSH: Hatha yoga for children. | Exercise for children.
Classification: LCC RJ133.7 .H45 2019 | DDC 613.7/046083--dc23
LC record available at https://lccn.loc.gov/2019013324

Printed on acid-free paper

This book is dedicated to the inner child in everyone. May we always remember to listen to that wisdom. Therein lies the joy.

Contents

Acknowledgments

The authors gratefully acknowledge the wisdom and support of Gail Silver, author and founder of Philadelphia's Yoga Child; our editor, Cathy Broberg; and the staff at Redleaf Press. We thank the kids and staff of all the schools and centers that we've worked with, especially The Giving Tree Daycare and Preschool in Philadelphia for allowing us to come in and photograph. Blessings to Shiva Das of Yoga on Main in Manayunk, Philadelphia, who taught both of us classical yoga and is the reason we met. Endless thanks to our families and friends for putting up with our busy schedules. And to our loyal dogs, Maddie and Cooper, and their best bud, Lulu, for being patient with us and keeping us grounded.

Introduction

Lila stormed into the room set up for yoga class. Anyone could see from her scowl—lips pursed, eyebrows up and drawn together—that she was hopping mad. She folded her arms in front of her chest.

"Ms. Sarah made me and Aiden stop playing our game!" she complained. "It was a good game, and we were following the rules!"

"Sometimes teachers have reasons for things, and we have to trust their reasons," suggested Ms. Sibyl, the teacher.

"I won't!" Lila shouted with a glare. But she agreed to sit in the circle and begin the yoga lesson.

"Put your hands on your belly. Take a deep breath in," Ms. Sybil began, leading the group in a slow, calm voice. "Feel the breath come into your belly. Now feel it go out, slowly, through your nose."

The group of four- and five-year-olds took five slow, deep breaths. Afterward Lila was visibly calmer, with her hands now resting at her sides. "I'm still a little bit mad," she confided to Ms. Sybil, "but I don't have to make that face anymore."

Can such a simple exercise really make a difference in the behavior and feelings of young children? In short, yes. It can. Yoga and mindfulness calm the mind, tame the emotions, and tone the body. This is true whether the body belongs to someone who is twenty-four years old, sixty-four, or four. In early childhood, yoga pairs two aspects of the whole child that we don't generally think of together: the emotional and physical. Yoga teaches children how to use the emotional and physical along with their breath to create a calmer, more balanced whole person. When you bring yoga and mindfulness to your classroom, you offer children a tool they can use to manage their emotions and work through conflicts calmly. These are social-emotional learning skills (often called SEL) that children can use anytime and anywhere

TEACHER TIME

You won't be able to create a calm classroom if you yourself are a churning sea of negative emotions. When you bring yoga to your class, your students are not the only ones who will benefit—you will too! By practicing yoga, you'll be better able to manage your own emotions and calm an overly busy mind, allow mental chatter to settle down, and bring clarity to your emotions so you experience less overall stress. As a result, you might find your friendships, family relationships, and work relationships becoming less challenging, allowing you to be more engaged in your classroom.

throughout their lives. Right now, today, they can put them to use in your classroom, creating a more harmonious place as they learn and play.

To be clear, yoga and mindfulness aren't magic. Your students won't suddenly become perfectly behaved or perfectly fit. Practicing yoga won't make anyone's life problems suddenly disappear. Some people will take to yoga more than others and experience greater benefits; this is true for children as well as adults. Even so, when people use yoga and mindfulness, they usually have an easier time taking life's difficulties more in stride. They are able to stay steadier and more centered in the face of everyday troubles. That, friends, is where peace and power lie.

WHAT ARE YOGA AND MINDFULNESS?

Let's begin by establishing what we mean by *yoga* and *mindfulness*.

Yoga is, in essence, a self-help program that originated in India about two thousand years ago. It includes movements (poses), breathing exercises, meditation, and other activities to help people achieve a sense of well-being and wholeness. In yoga the poses are linked to conscious, deep breathing. Without that link, poses are exercise but not yoga in the traditional sense.

In fact, the word *yoga* translates from Sanskrit as "to yoke," as when two oxen are yoked, or joined, together in a field to work. By yoking together the body, breath, mind, and spirit, a person can move through the world with ease and purpose.

Mindfulness is an ancient style of meditation. It involves paying attention to what is happening in the here and now without thinking about the past or anticipating the future. Achieving mindfulness can be much harder than it sounds for adults, as most of us spend surprisingly little time truly noticing the present moment. Mindfulness helps us learn to do this by teaching us to focus on things we usually ignore, such as breathing, the tension in our muscles, and the natural world around us, not judging or identifying them, but just noticing. Learning to do this for even a few moments can allow adults to find a sense of relaxation and well-being. Children naturally are better able to live in the present moment, but even a very young child who is upset, worried, or fearful about a situation at home or school may be distracted and unaware in your classroom. Learning mindfulness techniques gives children the tools to more easily manage their emotional upsets, empowering them to refocus on the here and now and more fully participate in the opportunities you provide. Over time, even children you think of as "difficult" may become a little less anxious and reactive to everyday challenges and a little more engaged when they learn these tools.

FACT-CHECKING BELIEFS ABOUT YOGA AND MINDFULNESS

Yoga and mindfulness are popular enough that they have entered the mainstream consciousness. But many people still have some misconceptions about both yoga and mindfulness. Let's explore a few of these inaccuracies.

Yoga Is Not a Religion

At least, it doesn't have to be. Yoga and mindfulness have roots in the religions of Asia, and many people who practice yoga and mindfulness in this country do so in conjunction with Hinduism, Buddhism, or other Eastern religions. For most preschool class-rooms, it will be appropriate to leave the religious aspects out. Yoga poses, breathing, and mindfulness by themselves do not have any religious content, and the instructions in this book do not include any—we use only English words to refer to poses and content (rather than the original Sanskrit).

Yoga Is Accessible to Every Body

Stereotypes about the kind of people who practice yoga exist, and like other stereotypes, they have a grain of truth but they're largely false. Yoga can be and is practiced by all sorts of people with all sizes and shapes of bodies. Yoga practitioners simply start where they are physically able and, over time, they improve. Not every person will be able to do every pose, and that's okay. Yoga poses can be adapted for each person's ability, including for children or adults with special needs. We'll talk about this much more in chapter 6.

Even Young Children Can Do Yoga

You might think the children in your class are too active or not focused enough to do yoga, but here, too, you start where they are. Young children don't need to be very calm to begin doing yoga; practicing yoga increases children's calmness! This book primarily focuses on children ages two to six. It is possible to do yoga and mindfulness with infants and young toddlers, but special training is recommended.

RESPECTING ROOTS

Depending on the ages and backgrounds of your students, talking about the origins of yoga may be appropriate in some classrooms. You could even use yoga as a starting point to explore another culture. However, you'll need to do so carefully and with sensitivity. In most cases, the place to start is with families in your class or your school who have Asian backgrounds and practice Hinduism or Buddhism. If it feels appropriate, consider asking them if they would be interested in coming to share with the group something from their culture that their child enjoys doing at home. (Keep in mind, though, that what they are interested in sharing may or may not be related to yoga and mindfulness. In fact, these practices may not be a part of their lives at all. Not all families from India are Hindu, and not all Hindus practice yoga.) If there isn't a family like this in your program who wants to come in, you could look to cultural groups in your area or personal contacts for help with planning appropriate lessons.

Teaching young children about a culture without the benefit of someone who represents the culture can be tricky. It's very easy for such a lesson to become a "tourist" curriculum, which is usually well intentioned but can come across as inauthentic and even disrespectful. For more on this, see the third edition of *Roots and Wings* by Stacey York.

Know that when you start bringing yoga and mindfulness into your classroom, it's possible that you will encounter resistance. Some staff members or students' families may be opposed to the idea. Some people may have a negative view of yoga or think that teaching it to young children won't work or is not worthwhile. We hope there is enough information in this book to help you convince them of its benefits.

In some cases, though, the objections may be religious. Families may be concerned that teaching yoga means teaching Hinduism or runs counter to their own religion. This belief is understandable. Yoga and Hinduism share the same roots, and some adult yoga studios incorporate aspects of Hindu practices into their classes and décor. Try to engage with families and listen to their concerns. Assure them that the activities you will present are about breathing and movement and are not religious in nature. Give examples of what you have in mind for their child's class so they can feel more comfortable.

Some families of Indian descent may have different concerns. Not all Indian families practice yoga, but if it is a valued part of their heritage, they may feel that a child-friendly version trivializes and disrespects something they hold dear. Again, communication and transparency are the keys to mutual understanding. Invite family members into your class to share their culture with your group. Ask if there are ways that you can incorporate yoga into your class that would feel respectful to them. You can even invite their help in planning or leading activities suitable for their children and the other children in the class.

In most cases, you and your families will be able to find ample common ground. Understand, however, that for some families, this matter touches on deeply held beliefs complicated by historical and political struggles. In some rare cases, compromise may not be possible. If you face this situation, speak with your director or other administrator to determine if yoga and mindfulness are a good fit for your setting.

USING THIS BOOK

This book begins by explaining in chapter 1 why it is beneficial to introduce yoga to young children. Chapter 2 outlines how to prepare for teaching yoga to your students and what, if anything, you'll need to do to make your classroom appropriate for yoga instruction. Chapter 3 delves into yoga breathing, including numerous breathing techniques to use with young children. In chapter 4 we describe yoga poses we recommend using with young children, along with the attributes they promote. Chapter 5 explores the various ways to use yoga with your students, including short "brain breaks" that can help with transitions, fun and games, and yogamagination sessions that enhance learning. It offers guided imagery activities and ways that yoga and mindfulness can support

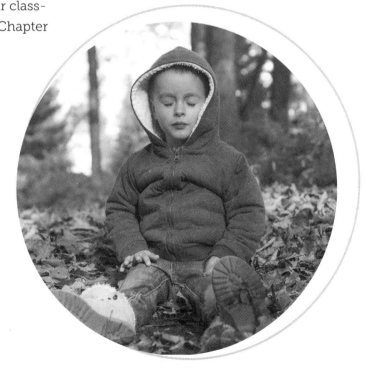

behavior management and social-emotional learning. Chapter 6 offers insights and techniques for using yoga with children of differing abilities.

Throughout this book we will be talking about yoga and mindfulness. To us these are not two different things. In the broad picture of yoga, breathing and mindfulness are included. So we won't repeat "mindfulness" each time we say yoga, but you will know we mean both!

We are assuming you already have some interest in yoga and probably at least a little bit of experience with it, but we are not assuming you are an expert. This book will offer you, as an early childhood teacher, the instructions you need to introduce yoga activities into your classroom.

CHAPTER 1

Why Yoga for Young Children

You may be wondering why you should introduce yoga to young children. It's a valid question. Research has shown that yoga benefits young children's learning, behavior, attention, and more, supporting them in so many ways (Mochan 2017). That said, yoga is only effective when children are engaged in the activity! Children reap the most benefits when lessons are age appropriate, fun, and relevant. Luckily, that's what this book is all about.

YOGA, MINDFULNESS, AND STRESS

One reason yoga is so beneficial is that it works in a physiological way to reduce stress. Yoga offers a way to handle feelings, become more self-aware, and establish a better relationship with the world and people around us. Less stress allows for greater mental clarity, something that supports classroom learning for young children. Who doesn't want to have a happy heart, healthy body, and calm mind?

The philosophy behind yoga considers people, including children, as having different layers, much like early childhood educators talk about the whole child. One layer included in yoga is the breath. Helping children become aware of their breath allows them to become aware of their state of mind. There is no doubt that the two are linked. When we are anxious, angry, or frightened, we may hold our breath and tense up our bodies. Stopping to take a deep breath can help us calm our bodies and realize what is actually occurring mentally and physically.

If you already practice yoga, you know the almost magical effects it can have on you after a stressful day. This is because yoga calms the nervous system. While it may seem like magic, there are physiological reasons why yoga makes people feel better, calmer, and more centered.

The effects start in the brain. A threatening experience activates our stress response, also known as "fight, flight, or freeze." This is our bodies' alarm system, notifying us about danger and prompting us to respond. (This used to be called only "fight or flight," but it has been changed because many people do indeed freeze, much like a rabbit in danger stays very still to avoid notice.)

This response is triggered when we perceive a threat, and a series of events takes place in our bodies and brains that allows us to respond. When we are in this state, our minds and bodies are on high alert. The threat is all we can focus on. We are consumed with an emotion, or many emotions, including fear, anger, anxiety, and so on. Whether the threat is real or imagined, the sensation in the body is definitely real. This response is the same whether you are a caveman seeing a saber-toothed tiger near you in the woods or a preschooler whose classmate is about to take a favorite toy. The emotions we feel overwhelm us. We are primed to take action, run, or hide—our breath gets shallow, our hearts beat faster, adrenaline (and other substances) kicks in.

When the threat is over, we can relax and go back to doing what we normally do. Inside our bodies, breathing, heart rate, hormones, and so on return to their regular everyday selves. This is a normal, healthy process. It's only when a person stays in that heightened state of stress that problems develop. For example, if children stay worried, their stress levels remain high, and they may suffer from what experts call "toxic stress." This may occur in cases where children live with extreme, long-term stress, including abuse and neglect. This degree of stress in children has been linked to impairments in learning, behavior, and well-being later in life (Shonkoff et al. 2012). In most cases, life doesn't have to be so extreme to be stressful for children. Many things can trigger the nervous system's stress response, including fear of not being accepted, being overwhelmed by a new environment, peer pressure, or new situations, to name a few.

Children will outgrow some of these as they get older, but some they won't. Yoga teaches children to become aware of their emotions and gives them strategies to calm themselves when they are feeling stressed. This often helps them feel better and respond better to the world. Yoga can help pull the nervous system out of that fight, flight, or freeze state and into peaceful relaxation.

YOGA AND LEARNING

Humans, especially very young humans, are not meant to sit for long periods of time. When children sit still for too long, the mind begins to turn off and the body stagnates. Today's children often are not able to spend many hours playing freely, and the consequences show. Many teachers are noticing that children's motor skills may not be as developed as those of previous generations. They need help from us as educators to reach their milestones.

Movement also enhances learning. It allows children to link concepts and experiences. When young children recognize just how an experience feels in their developing bodies, they form a meaningful connection between their inner self and the outer world. That connection leads to understanding—the brain is stimulated, neural pathways are developed, and cognition is enhanced.

Yoga is potentially one of the best tools to support physical and cognitive growth. It is also excellent for social-emotional growth because it helps reduce stress and helps children focus on their internal states.

Physical Learning

Yoga offers specific activities for physical development that are age appropriate, classroom appropriate, noncompetitive, and most definitely fun! Yoga activities for preschoolers are structured and generally done indoors. They do not replace unstructured outdoor play but offer other advantages to your class. With the range of yoga activities available, you can choose specific skill sets you want your class to work on. For example, many children today lack core strength. By working Silly Seal pose (page 64) into your yoga activities, you can support that critical development. Balance is another skill that is challenging for many preschoolers. Have your class try Tree pose (page 70) or Stork (page 67) every week, and watch them improve over time. (More significantly, your children will notice their own improvement.) You can do the same thing to encourage other important physical development skills. Yoga poses involve the whole body moving in different, sometimes unexpected ways, so poses encourage agility, flexibility, body awareness, and coordination. Chapter 4 will help you decide which poses to include for different aspects of physical learning.

Just like with social-emotional and cognitive learning, yoga activities aimed at physical development can work for all the children in your class. If a child in your group is having particular trouble with balance, for example, you can introduce a group balance activity and help everyone develop this skill.

Cognitive Learning

The actual stated purpose of yoga from *The Yoga-Sūtra of Patañjali*, one of the central texts about yoga, is to "calm the disturbances of the mind." In classroom terms, this means yoga contributes to the learning objectives of increased attention, concentration, and focus. The goals are achieved with activities such as paying attention to your own breathing, meditative walks, or practicing balance poses. All children can improve on these skills, including young children with attention and sensory issues.

The yoga activities we describe in this book also tap into and extend children's imaginations. Individual poses ask children to imagine how it feels to be a roaring lion, a starfish sunning itself on a rock, or many other animals or parts of nature. In chapter 5 we tell you how to put the poses together into "yogamagination" themes, extending the pretend aspects of the activity. You can ask children to pretend they are visiting a zoo, walking through a rain forest, or riding on a cloud.

We will offer suggestions for building yogamaginations to enhance the more academic aspects of your curriculum too. Using poses to act out how a caterpillar grows into a butterfly gives children a kinesthetic experience of this process. The same is true of imaginary activities, such as a walk through a spring meadow or a day at the beach.

Social-Emotional Learning

A relaxed, healthy child (or adult) is in a better state to learn and get along with others. Through planned activities and many teachable moments throughout your day, yoga can help children learn self-awareness and self-management. Taking time to focus on breathing allows children the time and space they need to tune in to themselves. This gives them the chance to distinguish which emotions they are feeling and to problem solve the best ways to act on those emotions. Once this self-regulation takes place, children are more ready, willing, and able to interact appropriately with peers and adults. They will be more capable of communicating their feelings and ideas and better able to resolve conflicts in socially acceptable ways that make sense to them.

One of the best things about yoga is that it has the potential to help every child. The practice offers a way for children, from the preschooler who enters your room with well-developed social and emotional skills to the one who seems overwhelmed by any conflict or transition, to develop and enhance their skills.

In our ever-changing world, we need to draw empathy, awareness, and connection into our classrooms. These qualities have roots in children's growing abilities to recognize their own emotions and how those emotions affect them. Young children often experience emotion without truly realizing what that sensation is inside of them. Emotions such as anger, frustration, fear, or anxiety can cause children to act out, using their bodies. A preschooler who is angry may throw a block at another child. One who is frightened may lash out verbally or simply withdraw, sometimes hiding in a cubby. Children can become overwhelmed by many things that adults may overlook.

Yoga can help children connect more directly with their own emotions and relate to others' feelings in more empathetic ways. The directed movement of yoga allows children (as well as adults) to release pent-up emotions in a controlled manner and recognize how emotions feel in their bodies. When they can identify how something truly feels for them, this sets the stage for recognizing how it might feel for someone else. Sharing this experience helps them connect the dots between mind, body, and emotion.

Yoga and mindfulness are tools that can allow children to separate their emotions from their bodies so they don't feel the need to act out. Understanding their own emotions helps children have a better handle on the ways they interact with their classmates, teachers, and families at home. Put another way, yoga and mindfulness help children develop social-emotional learning. With a better sense of self-awareness—the relationship between their minds, bodies, and emotions—they are better able to develop self-regulation and display responsible decision-making. A study reported in the *Journal of Child and Family Studies* in 2015 showed the effectiveness of a mindfulness-based yoga intervention in promoting self-regulation among preschool children ages three to five. A teacher used a mindfulness movement program (one description of yoga) throughout the school year. Increased self-regulation, longer attention spans, and the ability to delay gratification were among the significant effects observed (Razza et al. 2015). From this grows greater social awareness and control, which leads to greater ability to develop relationship skills.

TEACHER TIME

You are the central piece in the endeavor to develop social-emotional learning in your students. As you demonstrate the attributes of calm, thoughtful control that yoga cultivates, the children will begin to emulate you. In this way, your demeanor will coregulate the emotional temperatures of both your students and your classroom.

As the children in your room develop in these critical ways, you will begin to experience a more peaceful, aware, and connected environment in your room. The effect can even ripple out to the children's families and communities.

CHAPTER 2

Introducing Yoga into Your Classroom

To bring the benefits of yoga and mindfulness into your classroom, your first role is to create and hold space to facilitate students' self-exploration and learning. This chapter describes ways to make sure your yoga sessions are safe and comfortable. Your second role is to introduce and model the yoga. We'll get into that in later chapters.

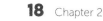

YOGA WITH YOUNG CHILDREN VERSUS ADULTS

When you think of yoga, what do you imagine? For most people, the answer is a class in a yoga studio or gym. A teacher leads from the front, and the students are adults who are highly motivated to work, move, and follow directions for a sixty- or ninety-minute class. The tone is serious, often quiet, and focused.

Using yoga with young children will be a bit different in numerous ways:

- The experience will be much less quiet and much more fun. Children's yoga uses animal names for many poses, and we commonly make sounds and hand motions to enhance the pose, roaring like a lion, hissing like a snake, or jumping like a monkey.

- During children's yoga, you will use themes and stories to tie the session together, engaging children's imaginations as well as their bodies.

- The instructions for the poses will be much looser, allowing for individual variation. You'll need to learn the various yoga poses so you can demonstrate them for the children and encourage them to copy you. Their developing bodies require that they do the poses in their own ways.

- Similarly, there needn't be the focus on alignment that exists in adult yoga classes. You will do much less correcting and paying attention to children's form. Avoid too many corrections, and don't "adjust"—that is, don't physically move their bodies into poses. Some children will be able to do poses more readily; some will have a harder time. All of them will develop gross-motor skills over time, including body awareness, muscle control and coordination, strength, balance, and flexibility.

- Classes will be shorter, and doing yoga with young children doesn't have to mean a class at all. Children's yoga varies from very short activities woven into the day to a dedicated yoga session called "yogamaginations" (thirty-minute maximum) modeled on an adult class but made appropriate for children. That might be what you had in mind when you picked up this book. You can also lead shorter large-group activities to facilitate transition points in your day. For example, lead a yoga exercise at circle time or when lining up to go outside. You can guide children individually through breathing exercises on an as-needed basis to help them learn self-control and enable them to respond appropriately to conflict and stress.

TEACHER TIME

If you are a fan of doing yoga but don't have time to attend a class, you still have many options for including this activity in your life. Adults also can benefit from doing yoga in ways that do not involve a class structure. Look online for short videos you can do in your living room, or create your own practice made up of poses you select. Once you know a few poses and breathing techniques, you can do them anytime and almost anywhere as you need them. Have stiff muscles when you wake up in the morning or after a long car ride? Do a few stretching poses to loosen up. Is your back sore after a day of working with children? Try a few heart-opening exercises that allow you to arch your back and stretch across the chest to provide a counterpose to the more hunched-forward position you've been holding. (Snake is a good option. You don't have to make the hissing sound, but you can!) Feeling angry or fearful? Take a moment for slow, deep breathing to help you soothe your emotions and reach a calmer, more collected state.

A primary distinction, of course, is the age of your students. Adults make their own decisions about attending yoga classes and have long ago learned how to behave in such a setting. Like in any other preschool activity, some of your students will be motivated to participate in yoga, while others will be less so. Some children will readily follow directions, but some won't.

In the following chapters, you will find different ways to use yoga in your early childhood classroom. Some of them will look much like what you think of when you imagine a typical adult yoga class. Others may seem different. They are all yoga! Remember that yoga is more than poses; breathing and even meditative activities are included as well.

Chapter 5 lists numerous ways you can incorporate a yoga program into your classroom. We suggest that you start small, with brain breaks and yoga games. This way both you and your children will become familiar and more comfortable with yoga activities. Once you have a few poses and breathing activities under your belt, you can move into yogamagination sessions, longer periods of yoga planned around a learning objective. Start small, but over time, you can expand the length of a session to twenty or

TEACHER TIME

Yoga in its full expression offers a rich set of practices and philosophy to help lead to a healthy, ethical lifestyle. The philosophy and practices together are called the Eight Limbs of Yoga. Poses are the third limb, and conscious breathing is the fourth, but there is more. For example, the first limb is a list of five things not to do, such as cause harm or be untruthful. The second lists five traits to strive for, such as discipline and contentment. Delving more deeply into this aspect of yoga is not appropriate for young children or for most school settings, but if you are interested in learning more or using yoga to improve your own health and wellness, consider consulting some of the resources at the end of this book.

twenty-five minutes for younger children, or up to thirty minutes for five- and six-year-olds.

How often to do any of these activities is really up to you. Many teachers like to do yoga on a weekly or semiweekly basis, sometimes as part of a rotation of "specials," like music or gym. Whatever schedule you choose, know that repeating yoga classes regularly allows children to become familiar with the poses and develop physical skills. While you can also reserve yoga for special occasions, this doesn't allow for practice and continued growth.

One important factor to always be aware of is that you are coregulating your group using your demeanor and the way you present yourself energetically. Children won't become calm and quiet if you are agitated. Model the ways you want them to behave.

Finally, children's yoga is a group activity. Yoga time can become "our" time, a time that encourages group unity among the children and you as well. Making sure everyone feels included creates a sense of cohesion and supports the children's journey into self-exploration.

TEACHER TIME

Have you ever walked into a chaotic classroom? The energy is frenetic, palpable. Your body picks it up, and you begin to catch the anxiety. This phenomenon is a two-way street: You know that if you come to class distracted or agitated, your class will pick up on that. The dynamics of yoga magnify that effect. There are no art materials, songs, or books to focus on. There is just you and your body. Getting started with yoga in your classroom means getting familiar enough with it so you can feel and project that calm, confident self. Remember to allow yourself the freedom to experience how the poses and breathing together feel in your body. Your children will feel the same. This is the magic of yoga.

THE BASICS

To enjoy the benefits of yoga, we first need to be sure that the children are safe and, second, that everyone feels included and seen.

Clothing

Clothing for yoga should be loose fitting. Most things that children wear will be appropriate. Shoes come off. On a floor that may be slippery, socks should come off too. Some children may resist, but it's not worth having a child slip. If you have a thick, textured rug, removing socks can be optional.

Space

Your own spatial awareness is key. Make sure each child has a spot with enough room to move freely in all directions without bumping into a neighbor. Once you have defined the space, look for potential hazards—cords, edges of furniture—and remove them. Explain what you are doing to help children develop their spatial awareness as well. If your room is small, consider pushing furniture out of the way or doing poses with small groups at a time.

Mats and Props

The good news is that mats aren't necessary! A circle-time carpet can work just as well. Marking each child's individual space is important though. If your carpet has letters, colors, creatures, or something similar along the edge, you can use those to indicate where children sit so they have enough personal space. If not, carpet squares or even a bit of masking tape on the floor can help children position themselves safely. If you prefer using mats, you can acquire them inexpensively online or sometimes from discount stores. Families may be willing to donate them.

Growing Bodies and Yoga

As we've discussed previously, in adult classes, teachers focus much more on proper alignment. With young children, we don't. They are still learning about their growing bodies, and their gross- and fine-motor skills are developing at very different rates. Some children may not be ready to place an ankle or a shoulder exactly where an adult would in a pose. If we correct them too much, they may become frustrated. Instead, we focus on the psychophysiological experience—how great it feels inside when we move.

Yoga should never hurt. If children tell you a pose hurts them, believe them! Remind them often that if a pose hurts, they should come out of it and try it again in a way that feels good for their body. (For example, bending the knees a little bit is a good way to approach discomfort in a forward bend.)

You also may need to encourage the children to simply not push themselves too hard. In some poses, children may discover muscles they weren't aware of and haven't developed, and they may feel the effort. Children's bones, muscles, tendons, and joints are growing at their own individual rates, and strength and flexibility vary also. Not only that, but children are proportioned differently than adults. In most cases, their legs are shorter in relation to the rest of their bodies, so a stretch that feels great to you may be painful for them.

At a basic level, yoga should always feel good!

Managing Behavior

The two simple safety rules for yoga are to stay in your own space and no running. Yoga is a time for looking and listening. As the teacher, you may invite children's comments from time to time. Otherwise, it's eyes up and a time for listening, not talking. Your tools to address potentially challenging behaviors in yoga with young children are the same ones you probably use for behavior management in other parts of your classroom:

- Set the expectations for the children at the outset.

- Let the children know what will happen if they don't follow the rules. Most likely, this will mean a set number of corrections from you (whatever number is appropriate for your group).

- If the children still don't act appropriately, they may need to be removed from the activity. While it's easy to get caught up in the mechanics of teaching young children about yoga, remember to take care of the basics. Hungry or tired children or those who need the bathroom are not going to be able to focus well. A group that's too large can also be a distraction. If the children are having trouble paying attention and none of these basics seems to be the reason, they may need some quiet time away from the activity to think for the general good of the group.

Try to keep from focusing on the negative behaviors of children or constantly correct them. Instead, reward the positive. When you catch children doing something correctly, make eye contact with them and give them the reward of your attention and positive speech. Let them know that you see them for who they are. Yoga is about subtlety. When you speak with a soft and steady voice, smile, and use other body language to communicate your approval, you will reinforce your students' positive behavior.

By using language, you have the ability to recognize individuals with comments, such as "I see Jayla is feeling like a strong, rooted tree—look at those branches reach to the sky" or "Aiden, I see how well you are listening and sitting in Easy Peasy pose." For the child who struggles to be still, this really is a huge accomplishment. Your words bring positive reinforcement and recognition of the emerging skill, letting them know they are seen. You can also use words that recognize the efforts of the whole group to acknowledge behavior and at the same time foster connectivity: "What great hissy snakes I see!" or "Look at you all resting so peacefully."

Occasionally children have become used to negative reinforcement, so this approach may take some time before it is effective. In the meantime, use a hand signal, such as a peace sign or placing your hand on your heart, to remind children to refocus.

DEVELOPMENTAL AND GROWTH EXPECTATIONS

As their teacher, you already have a good idea of what the children in your class are capable of doing. The chart below shows how developmental levels generally apply with yoga. Of course, children's developmental levels will vary!

Age	Physical	Social-Emotional	Creative
Two- to Three-Year-Olds Two-year-olds and young threes may not be able to do more difficult poses like Airplane or L on the Wall. Keep the poses simple and build on the children's developing strength over time.	Bilateral coordination develops, and they are testing their bodies to see what they can do. They learn skills like hopping with two feet and are beginning to develop balance and muscle control. Create a safe format and support their discoveries so they are not afraid to try new things.	Gaining in independence, children this age want to show how they are growing. Allowing them to take "safe risks," such as trying new poses, with your support and encouragement fosters self-esteem.	Two- and three-year-olds are learning through exploration of their environment, their bodies, and how the two relate. Their poses may not look like you think they should, but they are creating and learning about what their bodies can do.
Four- to Five-Year-Olds Because gross-motor skills are growing and they are excited to try new things, children this age will be eager to accept more challenging poses.	They are becoming more proficient at gross-motor activities and planning. Fine motor is developing. Ask them how many ways they can move their bodies. Noticing and pointing out how they are getting stronger can support their growth as they develop new skills.	This age is about going boldly where they've never been! Self-concept is strengthening, and children are really venturing out and eager to try new things. Poses that were difficult are now becoming achievable. Expressive/receptive language is growing, and they are learning to recognize and verbalize their own feelings and recognize others' experiences. They will really start to connect to mindfulness exercises.	Four- and five-year-olds like doing things in different ways, experimenting, and becoming more aware through exploration. This is a time when making stories open ended, allowing them to create their own yoga journeys, will be thoroughly enjoyed.

CHAPTER 3

How to Teach Yoga Breathing

One of the best skills we can teach the children in our care is conscious breathing. The breath is used to cool the body and redirect, refocus, and regulate emotions. Yoga offers many breathing techniques that affect the body in different ways. Some breaths are used to heat and energize the body, and some are used as a release for pent-up emotions, such as anger.

HOW DOES YOGA BREATHING WORK?

To teach yoga breathing, it helps to know the mechanics of how the lungs work. Specialists talk about breathing happening in two phases: The first is ventilation, when air comes into and out of the body. The second is respiration, which happens deeper in the lungs.

During ventilation, air travels through the nostrils down to the throat, larynx, and trachea and into the alveoli, little balls inside the lungs that resemble bunches of tiny grapes. As this is happening, the diaphragm—a large muscular structure that covers the base of the chest cavity—moves downward, and the muscles around the ribs expand, making room for the lungs to fill up with air. On an exhale, the diaphragm lifts and the muscles contract, pushing air out.

Respiration is when oxygen enters the body and carbon dioxide is released. This exchange happens within the alveoli. From here, oxygen passes through the lungs into the bloodstream and around the body, affecting everything, down to the cellular level. By breathing better, we are better nourishing our whole bodies.

Ventilation and respiration are automatic, controlled by the brain without conscious thought. But there is also voluntary breathing, where we begin to pay attention and take some control of the breath to change our state of being.

While breathing is, of course, vital to our physical being, it also affects our emotions. Just as fear causes rapid, shallow breathing in the fight, flight, or freeze response, uncontrolled rapid breathing can trigger fear. Controlled breathing can promote calmness or positive energy, depending on how it's done. Following are breathing techniques you can teach to your class. Spend time getting acquainted with these breaths. Just like other curriculum areas, it is a good idea to know the material beforehand. Practice using the different types, and notice how they make you feel so you better understand how they can help your children feel.

BREATHING TECHNIQUES

In these activities, you will be using language to help children notice their breathing and how it connects to emotions. Try to support them feeling the breath all around, not only inside but outside of them. Ask them to notice in their bodies where they feel the breath and to place a hand there to make the concept concrete. Ask them frequently to pay attention to how they feel when they do different types of breaths. When you are not doing yoga, you can remind children to use breath anytime they struggle with emotions—to stop, take a breath, and step back.

Three rounds of each breathing technique are plenty when your children are first learning it. If you want, you can build up to five rounds over time.

Belly Breath

Purpose: To cool down, calm, redirect, refocus

Children can do this either sitting up or lying flat on their backs. Instruct the children to place both hands on their bellies. Explain that their bellies are like balloons and need to be filled up with air. Invite them to breathe in through their noses and, when they do, feel how the balloons in their bellies grow. Then instruct them to breathe out through their noses and feel the balloons get smaller as

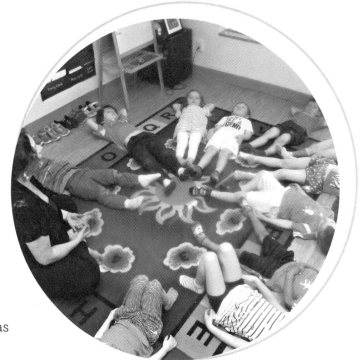

they deflate. Have them repeat this two or three times. Now have them move one hand up to their hearts. Invite them to breathe in and out through their noses again and see if they can feel their balloons grow all the way up to the hands at their hearts, then go all the way back down to their bellies when they exhale. Repeat this a few times.

For a more concrete experience, you can use eye pillows placed on their bellies to give added weight. (You can make your own eye pillows by filling child-size new socks with dried beans and lavender and sewing shut the open end.) The added weight brings a connection to the breath and also is a very grounding experience. This can be helpful for children who are anxious. A small Hoberman sphere (available online or sometimes in stores) is a great tool for demonstrating in three dimensions how the action of breathing happens. For interested older preschoolers, invite them to breathe in tandem with the expansion and contraction of the Hoberman sphere as you open and close it.

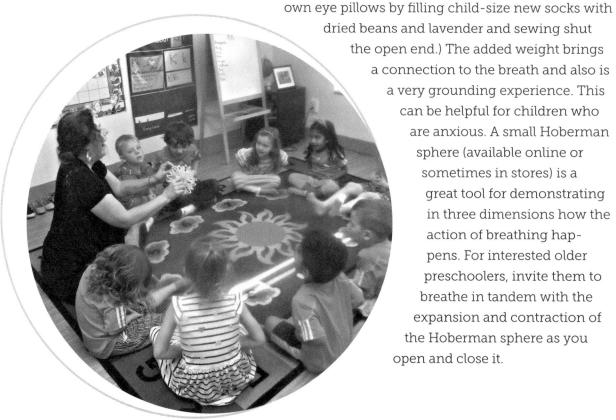

Open-and-Shut Breath

Purpose: To calm, cool, uplift

Invite your children to sit crisscross applesauce with the tops of their heads reaching up toward the sky (spines straight). Have them bring their hands palms together in front of their hearts, fingers pointing up. Invite them to close their eyes and think of something that makes them happy. As they take a big breath in, ask them to open their arms out toward the sides, and then, when they breathe out, to bring their hands back together. As they do this, remind them once or twice to think about their happy thing. This might be a family member, a special place, a pet, their favorite stuffed friend, or something else. After they have practiced this a few times, ask them to notice how they feel in their bodies. Children often are so externally stimulated that they don't get the chance just to be and to connect to their breath on this level.

Bird Breath

Purpose: To expand the lungs, create breath awareness

This pose is done seated. Ask the children what a bird has that helps them fly. Then tell them that for this activity, their arms will become wings. Invite them to reach their arms out to the sides with their fingers touching the floor. As they breathe in, they lift their arms up overhead, and as they breathe out, their arms come back down. As they continue this, remind them to bring their awareness to their breath to keep their birds up in the sky. After your children learn to do this, try adding another step: As they raise their arms, ask them to move their palms so they face up toward the sky. Then as they lower their arms, they should turn their palms over so they face the ground. Every breath helps their birds fly!

Slurping Breath

Purpose: To cool, calm, release anger

This can be done standing or sitting. There are two sets of instructions. You might tell your class, "There are two ways to do this kind of breathing because we are all different. Stick out your tongue and see if you can make a taco shape or a U shape with it. If you can, please do that. If you can't, put the tip of your tongue behind your top teeth." Demonstrate this. It might take a little while for the children to get comfortable with it. If you can't demonstrate the U, ask someone else to. Once everyone's tongue is in place, say, "Slurp in your breath, like you are drinking through a straw." Tell the children that this breath can actually cool them down like a cold lemonade, so it's a good breath to use in hot weather. Ask the children if their mouths or throats feel cooler after using this breathing technique.

Snakey Breath

Purpose: To cool, calm, release anger, be a little bit silly

Invite the children to do this either sitting down or lying on their bellies like snakes. Tell the children to bring their tongues up behind their teeth. Next, they should bring their top and bottom teeth together. Then ask them to open their lips and draw a breath in through their closed teeth. Have them "hiss" the breath out through their closed teeth. Repeat a few times. If the children are on their bellies, invite them to place their hands on the floor under their shoulders, palms down, elbows pointing up and back toward the ceiling. When they breathe in, they should "hiss" their snake heads up, and when they breathe out, have them "hiss" their snake heads down. Tell the children that they should be able to feel their bellies balloon out against the ground.

Bunny Breath

Purpose: To energize, create heat

When the weather is cool, you might want to use this technique before outside playtime. It strengthens core muscles and may make you feel a little bit warm. Ask the children to sit crisscross applesauce, or invite them to sit on their knees. Explain to them how bunnies breathe, wrinkling up their little noses and breathing quickly. Tell them, "We're going to breathe like bunnies." Ask them to bring their hands, palms forward, up by their ears to make bunny ears. Next, have them take three quick inhales through their noses, and then on the fourth count, let their air come out through their mouths (*in, in, in, out; in, in, in, out*). Let them practice a few times. Ask them if they feel warm in their bellies (most children say yes). The heat comes from using belly muscles they might not often use.

Buzzing Breath

Purpose: To calm, release anger, bring a smile

Invite the children to stand on their knees and then drop their bottoms back onto their heels. Have them take a big breath in and lift their arms up by their sides, like a T. They should make their arms very strong and straight. Then, taking another breath in and with their lips together, have them begin to let the breath out, making a buzzing sound like a bee. Tell them to continue until all the breath is out of their lungs. When that happens, they should bring their arms back in front of their hearts, palms together, and then do it again. Three times is plenty for this breathing technique. The children may tell you, "It tickles inside me!"

Dino Breath

Purpose: To release anger and frustration

In your own words, give these directions to your class with a lot of animation: "Imagine, friends, that you are a fierce tyrannosaurus rex. Stand with your feet slightly apart [demonstrate for them], take a big breath in, and lift your arms up high. When you breathe out, bend your knees, pull your hands into your belly, and let your breath go out with a big 'roar.' Take a big breath in, and do it again! Now, here's a special secret for you. If you're having a day when you're cranky, mad, or frustrated, try using this breath. It can make you feel much better." (Note: You may want to model how you want the children to roar when they release their breath. That way, the children will do it forcefully without losing control. If children scream, remind them that this is not a scream but a roar of breath going out.)

Wave Breath

Purpose: To calm or energize, depending on the directions you give

Talk to your students about waves on the beach, how they go up and come crashing down. Sometimes the waves are big and stormy; sometimes they are small and slow. Invite your children to stand with their hands by their sides. Tell them to take a big breath in as they lift their arms up overhead as the wave rises up. Then, as the wave recedes, ask them to fold forward and breathe out. This can be done at a slow and easy pace to calm and ground or at a more rapid-fire, stormy pace to energize.

Catch a Ball Breath

Purpose: To energize

Invite everyone to stand. The first time you introduce this breath, have children act out catching a ball in front of them and pulling it into their body. Next you can add the breath. Ask children to take a big breath in and lift their arms out in front of them to catch their big ball of breath. As they breathe out, they pull their ball toward their belly with a loud "Huh!" sound. Repeat this several times. You will find the children laughing while doing this and their moods becoming much brighter.

Running Breath

Purpose: To energize

This starts in Easy Peasy pose (see page 49). Tell the children to bring their arms, elbows bent, close to their bodies and move them as though they are running, breathing quickly in and out through the nose. You can vary it to run quickly or slowly, even up a hill to release excess pent-up energy. Note that you'll also find this breath in the Pose section. It works well as both.

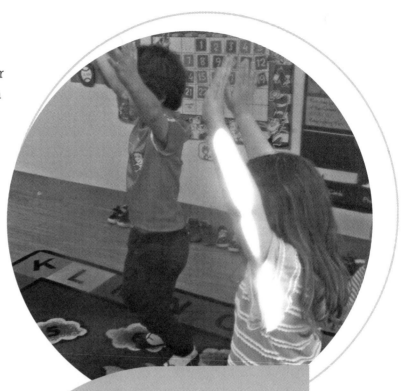

TEACHER TIME

Think of a time during your day when one or two of these breathing techniques would be useful to you. Remember that you can do these yourself at home, at work, or in your car—even in the staff room! Use calming breaths for times when you are angry or frustrated. Use energizing breaths when you're tired, after a bad night's sleep, or to get through a long week. Try to ignore any strange looks from the people around you. You may soon find them curiously interested and trying it out themselves.

CHAPTER 4

How to Teach Yoga Poses

Yoga postures originally came from ancient India and were practiced by sages. These poses were used to help guide the practitioner inward to a connection with body, breath, and spirit.

In traditional yoga, many of the names used for poses mirror things found in the environment, such as a tree, bridge, or chair. Other names are more like directions, such as forward fold or "stretch to the west." Today, thousands of years later, the structure and names of the poses in children's yoga can be more informal. You may even see different teachers calling the same posture by different names, and that's all right. The goal with children's yoga is to keep it fun and engaging so that they truly look forward to the practice.

THE EMOTIONAL ASPECTS OF POSES

When children move, they are also processing, experiencing sensory integration, and recognizing body sensations and emotions. A psychophysiological response occurs when children do poses, and the result is social-emotional learning. Poses can be used to help children recognize that their body position may affect how they feel. For example, they may feel less afraid when they become a Warrior or recognize that it feels good to be a Sparkling Star. You can help them tune in to these sensations using your language. When you give the directions for poses, remind them that they can feel brave like the Warrior, free like the Flying Bird, or relaxed like the Peaceful Piggy rolling in the mud. This helps them connect to the energy and attitude of the pose.

After children are familiar with a variety of poses, you can ask them to show you how they feel by doing their very own poses, right in their spots. Try this during your yoga session or anytime during your day. Showing you how they feel through poses can be empowering for children who may not be comfortable verbalizing their feelings. The child who shows you Fire-Breathing Dragon pose and says, "Guess what I am?" is telling you his or her exact state of being at that moment!

Comment on the progress the children make over time. When they are more experienced, you can remind them how at the beginning they all had a hard time with a pose, but now they can do it so well! Recognizing how they have grown together sets the tone for yoga to become a collective time.

THE PHYSICAL POSITIONS OF POSES

Yoga poses can be categorized by the positions or the motions they involve. Knowing the attributes of different poses can help you meet your goals for your students. By choosing specific poses in set categories, you can help children develop mentally, physically, and emotionally in a way that is not only healthy but a lot of fun. The last two categories, Just for Fun and Partner or Group poses, are not body positions but are enjoyable for children and foster group connections.

Foundational Poses

This book includes three foundational poses: Mountain, Easy Peasy, and Hands and Knees. They are poses in their own right but also serve as the foundation, or first step, for many other poses. Foundation poses create a strong, steady base.

Sitting-Down Poses

Many yoga sessions will start with these seated poses. They offer a sense of being centered, grounded, and rooted in place. They allow children to focus on the calm steadiness deep inside them, even when the outside world is not completely calm. For this reason, they are perfect to use when you want to help your students prepare for transition times in the day.

Kneeling Poses

A select few poses happen in a kneeling position, with children's bottoms on their heels. This position has the advantage of keeping the spine erect and allows the quadriceps to stretch. But it can be uncomfortable. If children have trouble with it, encourage them to try briefly, but then allow them to sit cross-legged.

Standing-Upright Poses

Often more challenging, these poses help strengthen growing legs, hips, and feet, as well as develop balance and gross-motor coordination. These poses require focusing the lower body down toward the earth and the upper body up toward the sky, bringing children a sense of connection and strength and power—roots and wings! A few standing poses are done asymmetrically, with feet pointing in different ways. Always do these poses twice, switching the position of the feet, so children get the same effects on both sides.

Lying-Down Poses

These poses bring rest and a positive sense of surrender. They allow children to really relax and feel fully supported by the floor and the earth beneath them. When children lie down at the end of the yoga session in Rest pose, their bodies are able to integrate the benefits of the other postures. Even very active children usually love the feeling of rest that comes from the Lying-Down poses.

Forward-Bending Poses

These poses are calming and help cultivate feelings of peace and acceptance. They apply gentle pressure to the digestive system (which may in turn promote healthy digestion) and allow back muscles to stretch, bringing release. On a day when there is a lot going on, the children are a bit fidgety, or you want to refocus the classroom energy, these poses are a great choice! Note that the purpose of these poses is muscular release, not to get their hands low toward the floor. Forcing a stretch can cause significant discomfort and possibly injury. Remind children not to push themselves too much while stretching. Many children will prefer to keep their knees somewhat bent when doing Forward-Bending poses, and that's fine.

Back-Bending Poses

These are energizing poses. They are a great way to cut through tiredness and distraction and wake up your group. They also open up the heart and can help children develop courage and reduce their fears. These postures bring flexibility and strength to children's spines. They also build core strength. Tell children to lift their belly buttons back toward their spines as they do these poses. Some children will find these poses very challenging, but remind them that their strength will build over time. Repeat these no more than three times in one session; one or two repetitions will usually do.

You may notice that children with a weak trunk area will bend their knees while doing these poses. This allows them to approximate the shape of the pose without relying on the core strength they lack. While this should improve over time, it gives you a picture of where they are now.

Active Poses

Active poses are defined by movement. They may be done in a variety of positions and combine different attributes of other poses. The same active pose may include elements of energizing, releasing, balancing, and strength building.

Twisting Poses

These bring flexibility to the spine and increase blood flow to vital organs when the twist is released. They are thought to help improve digestion, and they can also help clear the mind. Encourage young children to do gentle twists rather than deep twists.

Balance Poses

Balance poses are usually done standing. They help children develop poise and regulate their nervous systems, making their thoughts and bodies calmer and more balanced. These poses increase stability, improve visual and mental focus, and build confidence and strength. In all balance poses, it's important to remind children to make their bellies strong by pulling their belly buttons back to their spines and looking at one spot in front of them that won't move. (This means they shouldn't be looking at you or another child.) This will help them keep their balance. Tell them that when their eyes move, their thoughts and focus move, and their bodies will too.

Upside-Down Poses (Inversions)

These popular poses increase the blood supply to the brain. They can help young children develop confidence, reduce fear, and gain a different perspective of the world. That said, when working with children with special needs, check with family and even physicians before having them try these postures. Because of some children's unique physical conditions, certain inversions may do more harm than good.

Just for Fun Poses

We included this category for just that reason—fun. These poses bring play to your yoga session. Many of them include a big exhale, so they also offer emotional release.

Partner and Group Poses

Doing poses in pairs and groups helps teach respect and empathy for one another. Such poses also help build friendships among children and cultivate a sense of group cohesion. Wait to introduce these poses until the children are pretty familiar with yoga. Reminders to treat one another kindly and gently may be needed.

YOGA POSES

The yoga poses that follow are listed alphabetically to help you locate them. The descriptions include instructions for teaching the poses to young children and, in many cases, information about the physical skills the pose develops, the attributes and attitudes it helps convey, and brief tips and safety reminders where needed.

At the end of each pose description, you'll find key words in italics that refer to the physical position of the body and skills or attributes that the pose helps users develop. This information is intended to help you choose poses for your group that meet your objectives. The end of the book includes a special index that puts this information in one place for easy access.

Be sure to demonstrate the postures and give visual cues to help the children learn how to move into the positions. Use names for body parts, such as hips and forearms, to acquaint children with their own anatomy.

THE RELATIONSHIP BETWEEN YOGA, MINDFULNESS, AND NATURE

Thousands of years ago, sages observed and interpreted things in their day-to-day environment and then incorporated qualities from those things into yoga postures. They focused on ideals from things like a mountain, which is steady and unchanging even when things around it may not be, or a tree, which reaches for the sky while staying rooted in the earth. The more rooted the tree is, the less likely it is to topple over in a storm. Storms themselves came to represent emotions. By using yoga postures, both adults and children can embody the qualities of nature. Moving into the postures allows us to still and quiet the mind and connect to the seasons, elements, and broader world around us. This supports the development of understanding and empathy of others and ourselves.

Airplane

Instruct the children to stand with their feet together, like in Mountain pose (see page 56), but this time they are airplanes about to take off. Have them breathe in and lift their "wings" straight out from their shoulders. When they breathe out, they should bend at their bellies, keeping their backs flat. Then they breathe in and slide one foot back, keeping their toes touching the floor for balance. Ask the children to hold here for two or three breaths and imagine they are flying. Then instruct the children to breathe in, lifting their arms up over their heads and straightening their bodies to a standing position at the same time. Encourage them to feel the sun on their wings. Then tell them it's time to prepare for landing. They should breathe in, drop their wings back out, bend at their bellies, and slide the other leg back. Repeat the same process on this side. *Standing. Balance.*

Bug

Have the children lie on their bellies. Ask them if they've ever seen cicadas or locusts that often appear in the summer. Tell them that the Bug pose involves pretending they are cicadas. Have them bring their hands down alongside their bodies and bring their foreheads onto the ground. They should pull their belly buttons toward their spines, and as they take a deep breath in, they're going to lift their heads and hearts. Tell them to let out a "hmm" sound as they breathe their heads and hearts down. (You can also call this pose Flying Superman. Give the same directions but tell children they are superheroes flying above the ground.) To make this more challenging, have the children lift their legs at the same time as they lift their arms. This feels more like flying! *Belly. Energizing.*

Butterfly-Flutterby

Pretending to be butterflies is especially fun to do in the spring-time, but you can do it anytime! Have the children sit on their bottoms with the soles of their feet together and their knees out toward the side. Ask them to hold their feet with their hands and gently bounce, or butterfly, their knees up and down. Their legs create the butterfly's wings as it flies! Note that some children's knees will naturally reach the ground, while other children's knees will stay much higher. This difference is due to variations in anatomy. Let children know that however they do it is fine as long as it doesn't hurt. *Seated. Active.*

Caterpillar

The Caterpillar pose is very nice to do in the spring or anytime your students are experiencing growth and change. Explain to the children that we all start out very tiny, and then we grow! Invite them to lie down on their backs and pull their knees tightly into their bellies. Ask them to be very, very still because they are now caterpillars inside cocoons. Have them hold the position for a few breaths. Then tell them that something very magical is about to happen! Encourage them to start rocking side to side on their backs in their cocoons, and explain that they are about to pop out of their cocoons as brand-new butterflies! Now invite them to try out their new wings. To do this, they move their arms and legs away from their bodies and stretch them wide, taking care not to bump the person next to them. They can lower their legs and arms toward the floor then raise them again, still wide but stretched toward the ceiling. This is challenging to core strength, so they probably will only fly for a very short time. If you like, you can ask them to whisper the colors of their wings. *Back. Active.*

Caterpillar Coaster

The Caterpillar Coaster is a movement for a group to do together, but you know your students best. Some might take this as an invitation to misbehave. If you think it's appropriate for your group, it's a lot of fun and encourages group bonding. Be sure to give clear directions. Have the children line up in order of height, tallest in back and smallest in front. Tell the children at the two ends that they have the important jobs of leaders, and ask them to help by listening carefully to the instructions. Have all the children sit on the floor in their height-order row, each child facing the back of the person in front of him or her, legs out wide to the sides. They should be almost, but not quite, sitting in one another's laps. Now ask them to put their hands gently on the shoulders of the child in front of them. Tell the children that they are now a kiddie roller coaster. When they take a big breath in, the kiddie coaster is going *uuppp* the track. To make this happen, they all lean back together. When they breathe out, their kiddie coaster goes *dowwwn* the track as they all fold forward. This is suitable for older preschoolers, and you will need to help. *Seated. Group Pose.*

Chair

Have the children stand up with their feet shoulder-width apart and side by side like railroad tracks. When they breathe out, have them bend their knees and push their bottoms back and down while still standing. (Their bottoms don't touch the ground.) They can pretend they are sitting in an imaginary chair! When they breathe in, have them lift their arms up above their head, knees still bent. (Many children will straighten their legs at this point; just remind them gently to stay in the chair position.) After a moment, invite them to stand up on an in breath. This is challenging, so one repetition is enough. *Standing. Strength.*

Coat Sleeves

This is a fun pose that allows some freedom of movement. Use it as a morning wakeup or to release tension. Begin in a fairly relaxed Mountain pose (see page 56). Tell the children to imagine a coat hanging on a hanger. If you twist the hanger back and forth, the sleeves will flop forward and back. (Demonstrate with a coat if you'd like.) Direct the children to keep their feet planted on the floor and begin to twist their bodies right and left, letting their arms dangle. As they move, their arms will begin to flop forward and back. Children can do this as fast or as slow as they like. Make sure everyone has plenty of personal space to let their arms fly. *Standing. Twist.*

Cow/Kitty

The Cow/Kitty pose is about moving the spine. Cow pose stretches the mid-spine toward the floor, and Kitty stretches it toward the ceiling. Doing this pose involves going back and forth between these two positions. Have the children begin with their hands and knees on the ground. When they breathe in, they should let their bellies hang down toward the floor and lift their heads and tailbones up toward the ceiling. As they do this, they can let out a soft "moo" like a cow. Next, have them breathe out, lift the middles of their backs toward the ceiling, and let their heads and tailbones drop toward the floor, like a cat when it is frightened. Now they can give a soft "meow." *Hands and Knees. Active.*

Crocodile in the Mud

Invite the children to lie on their bellies with their arms bent at the elbow in front of them, one hand on top of the other. Have them place their foreheads on their hands. Ask them to feel their bellies move up and down while they breathe. Encourage them to be very quiet crocodiles as they rest in the cool, cool mud. *Belly. Calming.*

Double W

Have the children sit facing one another in pairs, with their knees facing the ceiling, feet on the floor. They should clasp their hands around one another's forearms. Their joint arms serve as bumpers to keep their knees inside. To begin, have the children place their heels on the floor and touch their toes to their partner's toes. You can stop here if you like. If your group is up for more of a challenge, have them press their feet into their partner's feet and begin to straighten their legs so their feet move toward the ceiling. To make this work, they will need to lean back a bit, lifting the heart. In the complete pose, their legs and bodies make a W shape. *Seated. Partner Pose.*

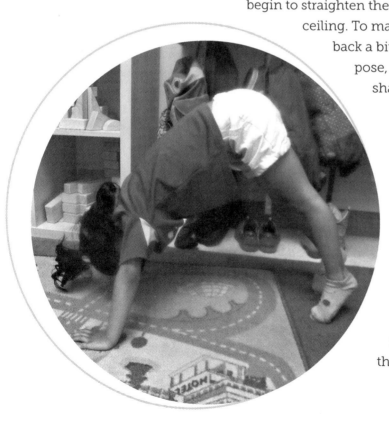

Downward Dog

Downward Dog is a lot of fun and a pose children are already likely to be familiar with. Start out standing. Instruct the children: "Take a big breath in, lift your arms up, and bend forward at your belly until your hands are on the ground. Now take two steps back with your feet." (Don't advise them to keep their feet flat on the floor once they have stepped back. Most children—or adults—will not be able to do this.) Many children lift their heads to see, so remind them to let their heads hang down without touching the ground. Their "dogs" can wag their tails by bending one knee at a time. To come out of the pose, children can bend their knees to the ground. *Hands and Feet. Inversion.*

Easy Peasy

This is the go-to seated pose for yoga. It is the same as crisscross applesauce or pretzel—children sit on their bottoms with their backs straight up, knees bent out to the side, ankles crossed. *Seated. Foundational.*

Feel the Breeze

Like Coat Sleeves (see page 47), Feel the Breeze also allows some freedom of movement and can be used to ener- gize or release pent-up steam. Have the children start in Mountain pose (see page 56). Then instruct them to breathe in and bring their arms up over their heads. Ask them to imagine that they are trees and their breath is the wind. As they breathe, invite them to move their arms side to side like branches swaying in the breeze. *Standing. Twist.*

Fire-Breathing Dragon

Start in a seated position. Have the children close their eyes and rub their hands together back and forth or in a circle. Ask them if they feel their dragon fire heat rising in their hands. Have them place their warmed-up hands onto their bellies. Tell them to breathe in and then breathe out with a brief, deep, sharp "Ha!"

sound. As they make the "Ha!" their belly buttons pull back toward their spines. Ask them to imagine the dragon fire releasing out of their mouths! (If the "dragons" are feeling angry, this is a great way to let it go.) With their hands still flat on their bellies, have them inhale and feel the bellies grow, then release the breath again with another "Ha!" Repeat this three times at most for young children. *Seated. Just for Fun.*

Flying Bird

Instruct the children to stand in Mountain pose (see page 56) and, with a breath in, lift their arms out to the sides from their shoulders, fingers outstretched. Have them sway their upper bodies, lifting one arm up as the other goes down, tipping from side to side. Repeat as often as you like. Then ask them to inhale and lift both arms up above their heads, then exhale and lower them down, bringing them to rest at their sides as they come in for a landing. *Standing. Strength (core).*

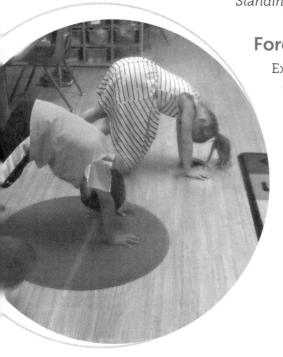

Forest

Explain to the children that trees are much stronger when there is a whole group of them. (Their roots interconnect, and some believe the trees even communicate!) Have the children stand in a circle. Refer to Tree pose (see page 70) for the basic instructions on the beginning pose, and demonstrate. Once they raise their arms as branches, have them touch fingertips with the children on either side of them. Remind them to be gentle and just touch, not grab. Now they are a forest of connected trees. *Standing. Group Pose.*

Giraffe

Start in a standing position, reminding your students that giraffes have very long legs and necks. Instruct the children to breathe one arm up and bend the wrist, with the other arm remaining by their sides. The upraised arm is the giraffe's long, long neck. Have them rotate the wrist around gently, pretending to be the giraffe's head looking around at the trees. Be sure to repeat on both sides. For an added challenge for older children, invite them to stay steady and come up on their tiptoes. *Standing. Balance.*

Go for a Walk

The goal of Go for a Walk is to have the children cross the midline. This is a developmental skill that some two-year-olds (and some older children) may not be ready to do. Start by standing in a circle. Say, "Let's walk to . . . ," and suggest an imaginary place, perhaps the park or a friend's house. Demonstrate bending one knee up and breathing in while bringing your opposite hand to it. Breathe out, return the hand and knee to the starting position, and switch sides. (Individual children may have trouble with this. Consider standing behind them and helping them get started so they can experience the movement pattern. Also note that while some children will be able to bring hand and knee together, others may just reach their thigh. And that's okay!) *Standing. Active.*

Gorilla

Invite the children to stand with their feet close together with a little space between, like railroad tracks. When they breathe in, ask them to bend at the belly and breathe out. They can sway their arms loosely side to side. They can also walk in this position. *Standing. Calming.*

Gorilla Tapping

Gorilla Tapping can be done seated or standing. The goal of this movement is to gently stimulate the thymus gland, a small gland that sits behind the breastbone, which is thought to invigorate the immune response. This works for adults too, but it's especially powerful for children. Consider adding this to your day during cold season. Demonstrate placing the fingertips of both hands right onto the breastbone and gently tapping, one hand after the other. To make this more fun, have the children take a big breath in and release it while making a humming sound, such as "ooh," "aah," or any vowel sound. When their breath is fully released, they are finished, so this will only take a short time. You can repeat it two or three times, perhaps changing the vowel sound with each repetition. *Seated or Standing. Just for Fun.*

Hands and Knees

This is the foundational position for poses done on all fours. Have the children place their hands, knees, and the tops of their feet on the ground in a comfortable manner. To make this a strong, solid foundation, their wrists should be in line with their shoulders, and their knees should be in line with their hips. Instruct them to position their fingertips so they are pointing forward. *Hands and Knees. Foundational.*

Hop to It (Frog/Bunny/Monkey)

Come down into a squat with your hands on the ground and invite the children to join you. Take a big breath in together and then jump! The exhale occurs very naturally when the children land. This pose can be a bunny, frog, or monkey, and it is a great way to divert excess energy! *Hands and Feet. Active.*

Horse

Horse is a fun, invigorating pose with active movement. That said, special awareness is key to make sure the children don't kick one another. Instruct the children to start out in Downward Dog, and as they press into their hands, they kick their legs up off the ground a little bit (roughly six inches) with their knees slightly bent, like a bucking horse. *Hands and Feet. Active.*

L on the Wall

The L on the Wall pose requires an ample amount of wall space. It's a pose that develops upper-body strength, so it will be a challenge for some children, but it builds confidence as well as strength. The pose looks exactly like what it's called. Have children stand next to the wall with their heels touching the wall, facing forward. Instruct them to move into Downward Dog, but instead of walking their feet back two steps, they walk their hands forward. Tell them to press into their hands and then lift one foot up onto the wall, and then the other, forming an upside-down L. They should stay in that position for only a few seconds. Then tell them to drop their feet down one at a time. You might want to have them do this one at a time (or two at a time for older children) so you can be a spotter for them. *Standing. Inversion.*

Let It Rain

Have the children start by standing in Mountain pose (see page 56), and then inhaling to Tall Mountain (see page 56). For this pose, they are going to act out a gentle rain. When the children breathe out, have them fold forward and touch their toes, wiggling their fingers as they go to imitate raindrops falling. (Remind them to leave a small bend in their knees.) Tell them to inhale and stand. When back in Tall Mountain, they can pretend to tickle the clouds to make it rain and then breathe out and fold forward again. *Standing. Active.*

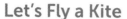

Let's Fly a Kite

Have the children begin this pose by standing straight and tall. Ask them if they've ever flown a kite or seen one flown. Explain to them that they are going to be using their breathing to keep the kite up off the ground. Invite the children to bring their palms together at their hearts and imagine what color and shape their kite is. Instruct them to take a big breath in and, with palms still together, lift their arms up above their heads, stretching and reaching toward the clouds. Have them move side to side as they breathe, like a kite moves with the wind. Once the children are familiar with this pose, you can suggest that they look up to watch the kite. Notice what happens—it's much harder to balance when you look up. *Standing. Balance.*

Lion

Lion is a great pose for releasing pent-up energy and having a fun time. It also stretches face and jaw muscles, where many of us hold a surprising amount of tension. Have the children begin by sitting on their heels. Then instruct them to place their palms on the ground in front of their knees—their lion paws— fingers spread wide. Ask them to take a deep breath into their bellies. They can release the breath by sticking out their tongues and making a "Blah!" sound so there is an audible release of breath. (We do not suggest an actual roar for this pose, as it can get out of hand. See Dino Breath on page 34 for suggestions if you want to use a roar.) Repeat this three times. Then suggest that they can go back to a regular seated position or fold forward so the lions can rest. *Kneeling. Just for Fun.*

London Bridge

Ask the children if they have ever gone over a bridge. Explain that a bridge rises up over water, highways, or train tracks so things can pass under it. Tell them that they are going to become bridges too. Have the children lie on their backs and bend their knees. Their hands and arms should be on the ground alongside them. Say, "We're going to take a deep breath in and lift our bottoms and backs up off the ground while we keep our feet, shoulders, and heads on the floor. When we breathe out, London Bridge comes down slowly." You can also say, "London Bridge is rising tall" when they come up. *Back. Strength.*

Mixer

This pose imitates the motion of an old-fashioned washing machine. Have the children sit crisscross applesauce or pretzel, and then instruct them to bring their arms out to the sides from their shoulders, with their palms facing up. Tell them to bend their elbows and bring their fingertips to touch their shoulders. Breathing in, they should twist their bodies to the right; breathing out, they should twist to the left. (Fingertips should stay on their shoulders.) You can instruct them to move quickly or slowly, or let them choose. This is an invigorating movement for the belly. Start with just a few rotations and build up to as much as thirty seconds. *Seated. Active.*

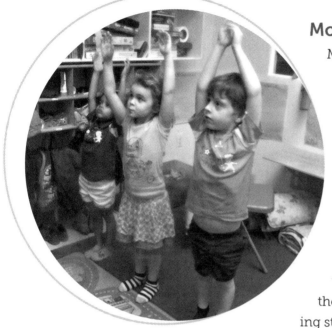

Mountain (Tall Mountain)

Mountain is a pose in itself and the foundation for all standing poses. It helps children develop strength, stability, and steadiness. Have the children stand with their feet pointing straight ahead with a little space in between, like railroad tracks. Their arms should be relaxed and their palms touching the sides of their thighs. Explain that their thigh muscles and especially their bellies are working, with their belly buttons trying to move back toward their spines. Instruct them to press their feet down into the earth and, while looking straight ahead, reach the tops of their heads to the sky. Tell them to imagine that if you were to go around the room and give them a nudge, they would be so strong and steady that they wouldn't fall over. You can stop here or, for Tall Mountain, invite them to take a breath in and raise their hands straight up over their shoulders. *Standing. Foundational.*

Ostrich (Wood Chopper/Elephant)

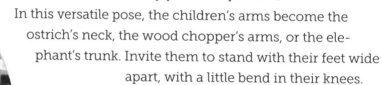

In this versatile pose, the children's arms become the ostrich's neck, the wood chopper's arms, or the elephant's trunk. Invite them to stand with their feet wide apart, with a little bend in their knees. When they take a big breath in, have them lift their hands up above their heads and put their palms together. Their arms should be as straight as possible, but many will keep a bend. When they breathe out, have them fold over and swing their arms side to side in front of them as they bend toward the floor. When they breathe in, they should lift their arms back up above their heads. You can repeat this two or three times. *Standing. Active.*

Peaceful Piggy

Everybody loves pigs! These piggies are very peaceful, and they love to roll around on their backs in the mud. Instruct the children to lie on their backs, bend their knees up, and reach to grab their feet with their hands. Their knees should bow outward, outside of their rib cages. Invite the children to roll back and forth on their backs in the mud. This pose allows them to give themselves a back massage and feels very nice and calming. If you like, on an exhale, have them softly sigh a long "oink." *Back. Calming.*

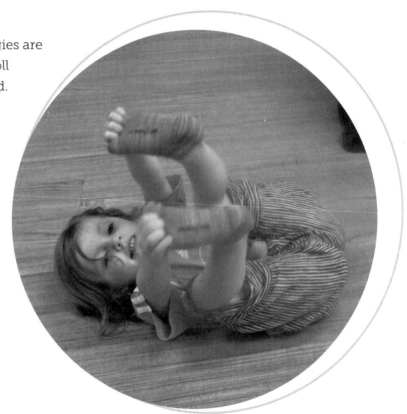

Rest

Rest is a very special pose that should always be done at the end of your yoga session. It can also be done anytime you want your group truly restful. It allows the body to absorb the beneficial effects of whatever other poses have been done. Invite the children to lie on their backs and place their hands on their bellies. Tell them they can close their eyes if they'd like to. You may find it helpful to dim the lights to create a quiet, calm mood. Every time they let out their breath, suggest to them that their body feels warm, soft, and at peace. Have them stay in this Rest pose for a while. One

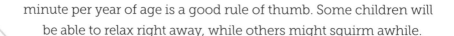

minute per year of age is a good rule of thumb. Some children will be able to relax right away, while others might squirm awhile. But even the most active children will eventually settle down. (You can use this time to calm yourself as well by breathing deeply. You will get the same benefits as they do and add to their experience.) While the children are resting, you can play music or offer a guided meditation in a soft, soothing voice. If the children are resting well, you can simply allow the room to be quiet. *Back. Calming.*

Ride My Bike

Invite the children to lie on their backs with their knees tucked in toward their bellies. Then instruct them to hold on to imaginary handlebars and begin to pedal with one leg positioned straight up to the sky and one with knee bent, and to alternate their legs as they breathe in and out. *Back. Active.*

Rock (Egg/Seed/Mouse)

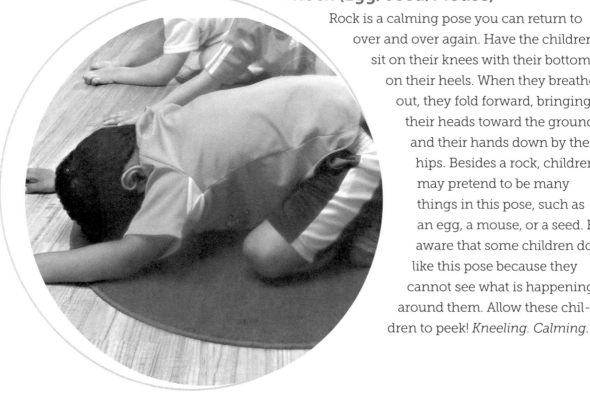

Rock is a calming pose you can return to over and over again. Have the children sit on their knees with their bottoms on their heels. When they breathe out, they fold forward, bringing their heads toward the ground and their hands down by their hips. Besides a rock, children may pretend to be many things in this pose, such as an egg, a mouse, or a seed. Be aware that some children don't like this pose because they cannot see what is happening around them. Allow these children to peek! *Kneeling. Calming.*

Rocking Horse

This pose is a relatively deep back bend and must be done with care. Some children will struggle with it, while others will find it easy and love it. It's better to save this until your students are more familiar with yoga. Have the children begin on their bellies, and explain that they are going to become rocking horses. Say, "What's going to make us rock is our bellies filling up with our breath." Have the children bend their knees and then bring their hands back to grab on to their feet behind them. Remind them to keep their knees close together and engage the strength of their belly muscles. Say, "When we take a breath in, we're going to lift up our heads, hearts, and legs by using our hands to lift up our feet. When we breathe out, our heads, hearts, and legs come back down to the floor. Because we're breathing, we're rocking! Breathe in and out a few times." *Belly. Energizing.*

Rope Pull

Have the children sit in pairs facing one another, legs outstretched in front of them, knees slightly bent. Then have them stretch their right arms out toward one another and grasp hands, with their left arms out behind them. When they take in a breath, ask them to switch the position of their hands, moving the left one forward and the right one back. Once again, they should stretch the unclasped arm behind their bodies and then join hands again. Repeat several times. This series of movements does many things. It reinforces crossing the midline, teaches teamwork, and encourages problem-solving skills. (It's more complicated to explain than it is to do! Once you and they understand the mechanics, this pose will be easy as well as fun.) *Seated. Partner Pose.*

Row Your Boat

Have the children sit with their knees bent, feet and bottoms on the ground. Invite them to bring their hands onto the backs of their thighs. Explain that they are going to make their bodies into boats. Explain that they need to make their bellies very strong and lift up their hearts toward the ceiling. (Be sure to demonstrate.) As you breathe in, rock back and try to lift your feet off the floor. Then rock forward, bringing your toes back to the ground. Rocking front to back, you can sing "Row, Row, Row Your Boat." This a lot of fun and builds strength, stamina, and concentration. *Seated. Strength.*

Run

The Run pose doubles as a breath and brings a lot of energy. Have the children start in Easy Peasy pose (see page 49). Then tell them to bring their arms, elbows bent, close to their bodies and move them as though they are running, breathing quickly in and out through the nose. It will really sound like running! *Seated. Active.*

Sally the Camel

Ask your students, "What does a camel have on its back?" The answer: humps! Explain that they are going to become camels and put humps on their backs. This pose is challenging for children because there are a few steps to get into it and it takes a lot of demonstration for them to understand. Have the children begin by sitting on their heels, knees bent. Tell them to take a big breath in and then rise up. (Their shins and feet stay on the ground, but their bottoms lift up so they are standing on their knees.) Once they are on their knees, instruct them to take a big breath in and lift their arms up above their head. When they breathe out, they should bend their elbows, bring their arms down, and place their hands on their backs. Say, "Look, friends, now we have two humps made from our arms!" To get out of the pose, tell the children to first lift their arms up above their heads, then breathe out, lowering their bottoms to their heels and dropping their foreheads down into Rock pose (see page 58). Bending their backs forward like this neutralizes the feeling of bending backward. *Kneeling. Energizing.*

Sandwich

Explain to the children that the class is going to have a picnic and they will make their very favorite sandwich. (You may have a child tell you he or she would rather have pizza—that's okay too.) Invite them to sit on their bottoms with their legs together out in front of them. Be sure that you demonstrate this and show them to keep at least a slight bend in their knees. Have them bring their palms together in front of their chests and think of their favorite sandwich. Suggest that they think about what goes in it and how it tastes. Tell them that their legs are the bottom piece of bread. Have them lift their arms up over their head, bend forward, and spread whatever they want on their sandwich. Explain that they might choose their sandwich filling to be peanut butter, cheese, or avocado. (Remember to have fun with this! If the children begin announcing their sandwiches, ask them to think it in their heads, but allow them to share a minute or two later.) Say, "Breathe in and come up, then breathe out and make your top half into the top slice of bread. Finally, rise up again with an inhale, exhale and bend, and pretend to eat your sandwich. Yum!" *Seated. Active.*

Satellite

Have the children stand with their feet wide apart and their arms outstretched, like in Sparkling Star (see page 66). Instruct them to take in a big breath, and when they breathe out, they should rotate their bodies to the right. When they breathe in, they should rotate their bodies to the left, holding their arms out straight. (This is different from Coat Sleeves, page 47, where children can let their arms swing freely.) If your group is up for the challenge, when they breathe out and rotate to the right, they can bend at their bellies and bring their left arms down to their right shins or ankles. Then have them take a big breath in to come back up to the starting position. When they breathe out, they should rotate again to the opposite side. *Standing. Twist.*

Scissors

Sitting in Easy Peasy pose (see page 49), have the children bring their arms straight out in front of them. Tell them that "X marks the spot" and to bring their elbows one above the other, creating an X with their arms. As they breathe in, have them open their arms away from one another, and as they breathe out, they should bring their arms back together again to make another X. As they repeat this, they should alternate which arm is on top of the X so the arms take turns. This will be challenging, but most children can do it with focus and effort. This is another pose that stimulates the hemispheres of the brain by having children practice crossing the midline. *Seated. Active.*

Sea Star

Sea Star is a nice pose for calming your group and giving the children an opportunity to rest. Instruct them to lie on their backs with their arms and legs positioned away from their sides, just like a sea star. Invite them to close their eyes and imagine they are lying on a beach. When they take a big breath in, they can imagine a wave washing up over their bellies, and when they breathe out, the wave pulls back. *Back. Calming.*

Seashell (Rolling Rock)

Instruct the children to lie on their backs and pull their knees into their bellies. Have them wrap their hands around their knees and rock gently side to side. The motion can be a seashell being rocked gently to sleep by waves in the ocean or a rolling rock. (The starting position for this pose is similar to Peaceful Piggy, page 57, but here the knees stay close together, while in Peaceful Piggy, they are out wide.) *Back. Calming.*

Seesaw

Pair up children who are about the same size and have them sit in pairs. Ask the students to sit crisscross applesauce with their knees touching their partner's knees. Then ask them to place their hands around their partner's forearms (being careful to avoid wrists and elbows). Now they will rock back and forth like a seesaw. When one goes back, the other moves forward, and then they both reverse position. Once the children understand the pose, you can introduce breath. The child who leans back breathes in, and the child who leans forward breathes out. To make this easier, you can have the pairs line up in a row. Direct all of the partners in one row to breathe in and lean back while all the partners in the other row breathe out and lean forward. Let the children repeat this a few times so they have a chance to understand the pattern. *Seated. Partner Pose.*

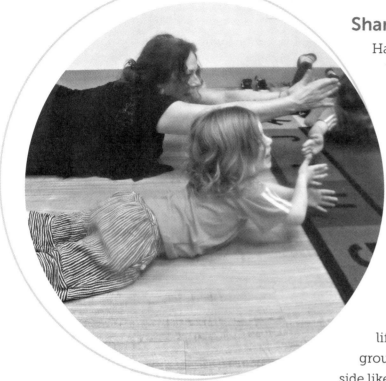

Shark

Have the children lie on their bellies, and tell them that they are going swimming in the ocean as sharks. (Children love this pose!) Have them bring their legs together and intertwine their hands on their backs. Their arms should be relatively straight but comfortable. Invite them to place their foreheads on the floor, and remind them to pull their belly buttons toward their spines. As they take a big breath in, they should lift their heads and arms up off the ground. Now tell them to rock side to side like a swimming shark. Their arms on their backs are the fin. *Belly. Energizing.*

Silly Seal

Have the children lie on their bellies. Say, "We're going to become silly seals. Bring your arms out in front of you on the ground and your legs close together, because seals just have a tail, not separate legs! We're going to take a big breath in and lift up our arms, heads, and hearts." Tell the children that as they breathe out, they can clap their hands together like a silly seal. This pose elicits many giggles and at the same time develops solid core strength. *Belly. Energizing.*

Slippy Slide

Have the children begin by sitting on their bottoms with their legs straight out in front of them. There should be a slight bend in their knees, and their hands go behind their backs, arms straight, palms to the ground. Ask them, "Do you like the slide on the playground? We're going to pretend to ride down. When we take a big breath in, we're going to press into our hands and lift our bottoms and legs up off the ground. Feet stay on the floor. This is how we go *up* the slide. [Demonstrate for children so they know to keep their legs straight.] When you breathe out, lower your body, keeping your arms as straight as you can, and we're going *down* the slide." Note that this is challenging for many children—and adults. It builds strength and stamina in the core and arms. Be sure not to lock your elbows. *Seated. Strength.*

Sloth

The Sloth pose is done lying on the back and is a fun way to cross the midline. Have the children lift their arms and legs straight up into the air. Then tell them to reach their opposite hands to the opposite legs, breathing in and breathing out as they alternate. Be sure to demonstrate this motion. The key is to move slowly, just like the sloth! *Back. Strength.*

Smell the Flowers

Seated in Butterfly-Flutterby (see page 45), tell the children, "Now we are going to smell the flowers, and they have lots of different smells! Take a big breath in, and when you breathe out, bring your noses toward your flowers [toes]." Some children will be able to reach their toes; many won't. Instruct them to inhale and lift back up. On the count of three, they can quietly share what their flowers smelled like. *Seated. Calming.*

Snake (Big Snake)

Have the children lie on their bellies and tell them they are about to become snakes. They should bring their legs together. Then tell them to bend their arms at the elbow and move their hands up until they are underneath their shoulders. Explain that snakes hiss, so they are going to use their breath to hiss and become a snake. Invite the children to drop their heads down and take a big breath in, lifting their snake head up, then hiss back down, rocking their bodies as they go. To transform a Snake into a Big Snake, instruct your group to lift their hearts and let their arms straighten by pressing into their palms as they take a breath in so their snake rises up high. *Belly. Energizing.*

Sparkling Star

Instruct the children to stand with their feet wide apart and open their arms out wide to the sides, straight out from their shoulders. To make their stars sparkle, they can open and close their hands. (This pose also makes a nice snowflake.) *Standing. Active.*

Standing House

It's important to match children with partners of similar height for the Standing House pose. Have the children stand facing their partners about an arm's length apart. Tell them to bring their arms up over their heads, keeping their elbows fairly straight, and touch their palms to their partner's palms. Their arms form the roof of the house. Next they step back a little bit, leaning on one another's arms for support so their bodies form the walls. For added support, you can have the children move to a designated wall and, still facing one another, each press one hip against the wall next to them. This pose teaches the importance of building a strong foundation and keeps children cooperating and focused on one another. *Standing. Partner Pose.*

Stork

Ask the children if they've ever seen a bird stand on one leg. Have the children stand up and pick out a spot on the wall to look at; this will help them balance. Instruct them to make one leg very strong and to slightly bend the other, lifting the heel of the bent leg so only their toes on that foot are touching the ground. Then tell them to take a breath in and lift their arms out to the sides like wings until their wings are up over their heads. They should try to hold this position for a few seconds. Then, on an exhale, have them lower the leg back down. Repeat this on the other side. *Standing. Balance.*

Stormy Weather

Have the children move into Chair pose (see page 46). Do it yourself and point out how your body is shaped like a lightning bolt! Now have them breathe out, bend over, and drum the ground with their hands. Remind them to bend their knees. This is thunder. This pose is a great way for young children to release pent-up anger and emotion and just plain make some noise. For a calmer version, you can do thunder from a seated position. *Standing or Seated. Just for Fun.*

Surfer

The Surfer pose starts the same way as Teapot (see page 69). Have the children stand with their bodies facing sideways, toes on the front foot pointing ahead and toes on the back foot pointing in a little bit. Tell them they are going to be balancing on waves. Instruct them to take a big breath in and lift their arms straight out from their shoulders. Have them look over their front arm, watching for the next big wave to come in. When you tell them it's coming, they should breathe out and bend their front knee. Have them take a few breaths while balancing, and then while breathing in, have them straighten their front leg. Say, "Now it's time to ride the surfboard home." Have them pivot so that the front foot becomes the back foot on the surfboard and the back foot becomes the front foot. Explain that now they are facing back toward shore. Again, have them breathe out and bend their front knee. Let them ride the imaginary surfboard for a few breaths. To end you can have them jump off their surfboards: Have them drop their arms down and pivot their feet again, this time so their feet face the side of the board. Now their legs are in the same position as they would be in Sparkling Star (see page 66). Tell them to exhale, bend their knees, and jump their feet together to jump off the board. *Asymmetrical Standing. Strength (core).*

Swinging

Have the children sit crisscross applesauce. Instruct them to breathe in and lift their arms up and away from their shoulders. When they breathe out, they should twist their bodies in one direction, arms outstretched. When they breathe in, they swing in the opposite direction. Be sure to demonstrate, because some children may have a hard time understanding the directions for this pose. Once they see it, though, they can generally do it. *Seated. Twist.*

Table (Crab)

Have the children sit on their bottoms with their knees bent and their feet and hands on the ground, fingers pointing toward their feet. Instruct them to take a big breath in and lift their bottom and belly up off the ground. This is how they turn themselves into a table! Then tell them to breathe out and drop their bottoms back down. (Note that young children won't be able to make their bellies flat like a table—they just don't have the strength. This is fine.) Thematically, this pose goes nicely with Chair (see page 46). To turn it into Crab, have the children walk on their hands and feet. *Seated. Strength.*

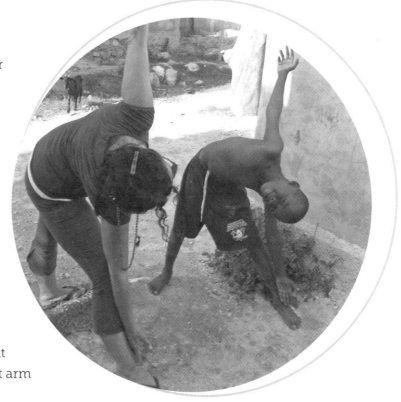

Teapot

Have the children stand with their legs wide apart and then move one foot forward so they are standing asymmetrically. They should have the toes on their front foot pointing ahead and the toes on their back foot pointing slightly out. From this position, instruct them to breathe in and lift their arms up to shoulder height. When they breathe out, they will be a steaming teapot. Instruct them to put their back hand on their hip to make the handle; their front arm becomes the spout. The front arm tips forward and then down to pour out the imaginary tea. Stand straight up again, and then put the opposite foot in front. Tip, pour, repeat! *Asymmetrical Standing. Strength (core).*

Tickle Toes

Instruct the children to lie on their backs and pull their knees up to their bellies. Tell them that when they take a big breath in, they're going to reach their toes up to the sky and imagine that they are tickling the clouds with their toes. *Back. Inversion.*

Tree

The Tree is a familiar pose to many people, but with children we do it a little differently. Instead of placing one foot up against the other leg, as you may have seen, for children the toes of the second leg remain on the ground. Have the children begin by standing with their feet like railroad tracks. Explain that trees have roots that move down into the ground to hold them steady, and they have branches that reach up toward the sky. Ask the children to close their eyes and feel their roots come out of their feet and connect down into the ground. Invite them to open their eyes and then breathe in and lift their arms up above their heads, like branches. Invite them to bend one knee slightly and turn it out toward the side, lifting their heels but leaving their toes on the floor. Ask them to look up at the sky and imagine the sun on their faces and branches. (Some children will want to try the adult form of this pose, but most will wobble all over. Encourage them to stay rooted and grounded, because we don't want our trees in the forest to fall over.) *Standing. Balance.*

Turtle

Tell the children that turtles carry their homes wherever they go, and when they become frightened of something, they can find calm by going inside their shells. Invite them to sit on their bottoms with their legs opened out to each side, keeping a soft bend in the knees. Have them take a big breath in and lift their arms up above their heads and look up. Then have them breathe out, bend forward, and close their shell by moving their heads toward the ground and moving their hands to the ground in front of them. Ask them to take a few breaths while inside their shell and then, on an in breath, lift their heads back up. Say, "Look to the right, look to the left. It's okay to come out!" *Seated. Calming.*

Warmth of the Sun (Moon in the Sky)

Warmth of the Sun and Moon in the Sky are the same pose. Instruct the children to start standing in Mountain pose (see page 56) and then inhale to raise their arms into Tall Mountain (see page 56). Tell them to let their fingertips touch above their heads, creating an oval shape that is either the shiny sun or the bright, full moon. With the sun, instruct children to feel its warmth. You can add a crescent to the moon by having the children breathe out and release one arm down to their sides. As they inhale, they move that arm back up and repeat on the other side. *Standing. Active.*

Warrior

Begin by having the children stand in Mountain pose (see page 56). Instruct them to step one leg way back and, at the same time, bring their arms up over their heads. On their out breath, have them bend their front knee. This is Warrior pose. Explain to them that they are peaceful warriors, strong, steady, and brave. After a few breaths in this pose, tell them that on their next breath out, they can step their back foot up to meet the front foot. Have them take a breath or two to rest, then instruct them to breathe in again and step the other foot way back. Repeat the process with the opposite leg forward. *Asymmetrical Standing. Strength.*

Wheels on the Bus

Have the children sit in Easy Peasy pose (see page 49). Tell them to bring their arms in front of them, one hand over the other, palms down. Ask them to focus on their hands and rotate their arms around one another, as you would do to sing "The Wheels on the Bus." Feel free to sing the verse if you would like. The goal here is for the children to focus their eyes on the hand motion. You can also add more verses from the song. Have the children raise their arms straight up toward the ceiling and, as they breathe in and out, sway their arms side to side for wipers on the bus. Last, have them bring their palms together in front of their hearts, elbows pointing to the side. When they breathe in, their hands open out to the sides like bus doors. When they breathe out, their arms/bus doors fold back in and their hands come together. *Seated. Just for Fun.*

Who Can Make a Rainbow?

Begin by having the children stand with their feet like train tracks. Invite them to breathe their arms up overhead and, as they breathe out, reach their arms and fingers to the side, making a curve with their bodies. Repeat in the other direction. They can also stretch to reach the friend next to them. *Standing. Balance.*

CHAPTER 5

Using Yoga in Your Classroom

Having reached this point in the book, you are most likely trying to figure out exactly how you're going to fit yoga into your classroom. Your mind already is trying to fit in everything else you need to cover during the classroom day without adding one more thing, but don't worry! There are lots of ways to use yoga that can suit different purposes. They all use breath and poses and benefit your children physically, cognitively, and emotionally.

The other thing all these strategies and methods have in common is fun! Young children learn through play; indeed, play is intrinsic to their learning process. It is their work, and it feels good to them. When you make the job a game, it becomes magic

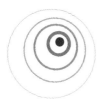

(it worked pretty well for Mary Poppins, if you recall), so we keep the "job" of doing yoga playful and lighthearted. This means for you too! Remember that you are not (most likely) a registered yoga teacher who has to have everything just right. Anything you do to start integrating yoga ideas and activities—as long as it's safe, of course—is going to help create a wonderful day and enrich your students' social-emotional learning.

This chapter explains various types of yoga activities, but they are really very similar. The differences are how long they are, when you want to fit them into your day, and what specific purpose you want them to serve. We'll start with the shortest type of yoga activity, brain breaks. These take just a few minutes and fit into your day whenever you need them. They are good for helping children come together at group times or easing transitions between activities.

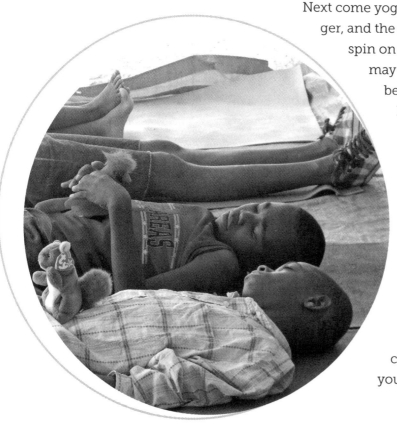

Next come yoga games. These are a little bit longer, and the focus is on fun. Most put a yoga spin on something you and the children may already know. Yoga games can be used in transition times if you have a little more time to fill. They're also great for rainy days when you need a fun, focused physical activity to help children let off steam.

Both brain breaks and yoga games are a good place to begin your classroom yoga journey. Since they are shorter, they will be easier for you to teach and for children to learn. They give everyone a chance to master a few poses that you can build on later.

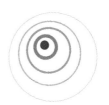

After brain breaks and yoga games are more complete yoga sessions, called "yogamaginations" because they combine yoga poses and breath with imagination. There are almost endless options for creating yogamaginations, and they can be customized for a wide variety of learning objectives. Once you decide on your objective, you choose which poses and breaths to include, sequence them in a way that makes sense, then lead your students in an activity you can all benefit from and enjoy. You can work on gross-motor skills or reinforce learning aspects of your curriculum. You can communicate yoga themes such as kindness or contentment. You can connect with nature and bring books to life. We offer numerous lesson plans to get you started, and then it's time for your creativity to soar!

Next are guided meditations. These are truly special activities. While yogamaginations feature plenty of action and movement, guided meditation is quiet. It is done either seated or lying down and invites children to turn their attention inward while you lead them on an extended imaginary journey.

The end of this chapter reminds you that yoga need not be done as a group or at a certain time. You can put yoga to work as a self-regulation tool anytime during your day if children need to maintain control of their behavior or regain that control when it momentarily slips away.

BRAIN BREAKS

Yoga activities can help ease transition times. Children are often reluctant to move from one activity to another, and this can bring up emotions. If not managed, transitions can become difficult, potentially setting your whole day on its heels. The first step is to make the children aware that a change of activity is imminent. You probably already have a warning signal, whether it's a song, a cleanup bell, or something else. These are often sufficient, but there is sometimes a child or children who may still struggle. This is your opportunity to use yoga.

Or you may have one of those days when you can tell that your children are beginning their morning feeling tired and lethargic, like they'd rather be home in bed. For times like this, you might want to get the energy up and have a little fun. Moving their bodies and using their breath can help uplift children and make them feel more awake and ready to meet their day. When bodies are lethargic, they tend to be cool. Energizing activities move the blood, make the heart pump faster, and generate warmth from within as they create mental and physical stimulation.

While yoga done as a class requires plenty of space, in yoga transitions, we adapt the type of movements done to the space available, so less overall space is required. In some cases, a yoga transition may include only breathing exercises, making any space adequate.

The brain breaks that follow can be used with a whole group or part of a group, depending on your needs. They can also be done occasionally or as part of a daily routine. Children thrive with con-sistency, so it may be a good idea to choose one for specific times during the day. That said, sometimes it could be fun to shake it up.

An example of an occasional part-group yoga transition would be one you lead with children who are lined up to go outside while they wait for the rest of their classmates to be ready. You could alternate the yoga transition with other types of transition activi-ties and games, either following a set weekly sequence (Monday is singing, Tuesday is yoga, and so on) or just as your or your chil-dren's fancy strikes. Note that this requires at least two teachers, one for the yoga activity and one to assist other children who are still getting ready. A possible daily full-group yoga transition could be part of your morning circle time routine, where children know to expect this activity every day. Consider your own program for other options.

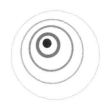

Here are ideas for fun brain breaks to ease transition times throughout the day.

Breathing Exercises

Remember chapter 3? Breathing activities in and of themselves are brain breaks, allowing children to reset themselves. Turn to some of these exercises to build energy, such as *Bunny Breath*, *Dino Breath*, and *Running Breath*, and others such as *Slurping Breath* to calm down. The guided imagery Happy Heart (see page 109) is another good choice.

Half Star to Star

Have the children stand in *Sparkling Star* pose, breathe out, and then bring their left arms to touch their right. Then have them breathe and open their arms back into *Sparkling Star*. When they breathe out again, their arms should come together on the other side. Repeat.

Reach the Sky

Instruct the children to breathe in and reach up, then breathe out and reach down. While they do this, say, "Reach up high, touch the sky. Reach down low, touch your toes." (Children should feel free to bend their knees to reach their toes if needed.) This is a good way to move energy with controlled breath and direction.

Single Poses

Doing just one standing pose that doesn't take up a lot of room or time can also be effective as a brain break. Good energy raisers are *Warrior*, *Chair*, and *Surfer*, while forward-bending poses such as *Gorilla* or *Rock* are good energy calmers.

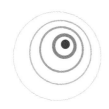

Stop, Drop, and Rock

When the energy level is too high or your group clearly needs a moment to regroup, it's Stop, Drop, and Rock to the rescue. Give the children the instruction to stop, drop to their knees, and go into *Rock* pose for a few breaths. When you feel the energy is lowered, let them know they can come up.

Twinkle, Little Star

Have the children stand in *Sparkling Star* pose and begin singing "Twinkle, Twinkle, Little Star." As the song is sung, they should twist and turn side to side with their arms outstretched. Have them breathe in and move their arms above their heads way up high, "like a diamond in the sky" with palms together and, when they breathe out, move them back down so they are straight out from their shoulders, and continue twisting.

Wiggly Worm

Have the children stand in one spot and begin to wiggle their toes, legs, arms, bodies, and heads until all of them is wiggling like a worm. Do this for a maximum of thirty seconds.

YOGA FUN AND GAMES

You might be wondering just how you are going to incorporate games into your yoga classroom. The answer is in a very fun and familiar way, using games that children may already know in new ways that incorporate yoga. They are a lovely way to bring movement into your class, especially on a rainy day when going outside is not an option. Because it's difficult for young children to remain still for an extended time, yoga games make a welcome activity. Games are a great way to promote learning, and children love to play them! The games you will be playing have multiple benefits—everything from gross-motor planning and crossing the midline to focus, enhanced listening skills, cognitive

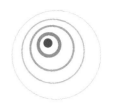

development, and recall skills. That is a lot of bang for your buck, as the saying goes. (Crossing the midline of the body is an important developmental skill that most children develop around age three. It is important for sensorimotor function. We address this in more detail in chapter 6.)

Note that the yoga games in this book are noncompetitive. If children start to compete, remind them that when they play and work together on the same team, they *all* win. The biggest rule here is to have fun.

The Bell Game

The Bell Game enhances auditory skills and focus. You will need a singing bowl or a Woodstock small chime. These instruments create sounds that resonate for surprisingly long periods of time. Begin by instructing the children to sit in a circle; tell them that they are going to be using one of their superpowers—hearing. Explain that you have a special chime and that it makes a special sound that goes on a long time until it is all the way quiet. Demonstrate the sound. Invite the children to close their eyes while you ring the chime. Tell them to put a hand on their hearts when they can't hear the sound anymore.

Clear the Clouds

The purpose of this game is to support and strengthen breath capacity while improving focus and motor control. All you need are straws and cotton balls; tissues work equally well.

Have the children start out on their hands and knees on a smooth surface like tile or a gym floor. Give each a straw (ones that are not flexible are best) and a tissue or cotton ball. Inform them that their breath is like the wind, and it can blow the clouds away. At your cue, have them come down to their cotton ball or tissue "cloud" and start blowing through the straw. Cheer them on as they develop strength and coordination! This game is a lovely add-on to a day when you read *It Looked Like Spilt Milk.*

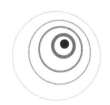

Going on a Bear Hunt

Is there is a child, or adult for that matter, who does not like to play this game? It's active, imaginative, and a good bit of fun. The more animated you are, the better! The purpose here is to work on crossing the midline, the sense of the body's position in space, and positional words. There is one part for each verse that goes "can't go over it, can't go under it." When you say "over," inhale the arms up overhead, and when you say "under," breathe the arms down on the ground in front of you as you fold forward. You and the children do the poses and arm movements together. For the words in italics below, have the children recite along with you. Instructions for poses enclosed in brackets are in chapter 4. Starting out with the children seated, the game goes like this:

"We're going on a bear hunt, we're going on a bear hunt, we're not afraid. I see a river. *Can't go over it, can't go under it,* guess we are going to swim through it [move the arms in circular swimming motion].

"We're going on a bear hunt, we're going on a bear hunt, we're not afraid. I see mud. Squishy, gooey mud. *Can't go over it, can't go under it,* guess we're going to walk through it. [*Go for a Walk.*]

"We're going on a bear hunt, we're going on a bear hunt, we're not afraid. I see a forest of trees. *Can't go over it, can't go under it,* guess we are going to go through it. [Each child moves into *Tree* pose, creating a *Forest*.]

"We're going on a bear hunt, we're going on a bear hunt, we're not afraid. I hear a breeze. *Can't go over it, can't go under it,* guess we are going to go through it. [*Feel the Breeze.*]

"We're going on a bear hunt, we're going on a bear hunt, we're not afraid. I smell a field of flowers. *Can't go over it, can't go under it,* guess we are going to tiptoe through it. [*Smell the Flowers.*]

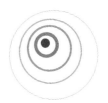

"We're going on a bear hunt, we're going on a bear hunt, we're not afraid. Uh-oh—I see a bear! Run! [*Run.*]

"Back through the flowers [*Smell the Flowers*], back through the breeze [*Feel the Breeze*], back through the forest of trees [*Forest*], back through the mud [*Go for a Walk*], back past the river [swimming motions], into our house, and into our bed. [Have the children sit down and place their legs straight out on the ground. Fold forward with hands going toward ankles, a slight bend in the knees. Breathe the arms up as you pull the pretend covers up from your ankles and over your head as you lie back.] Now let's rest!"

While the group is resting, call attention to their breath. Invite your group to place one of their hands on their bellies and one on their hearts, and then be as quiet as they can while they listen to their breath so the bear doesn't hear them. See if they notice their hearts beating quickly and slowing down as they rest.

Head, Shoulders, Knees, and Toes

This version of Head, Shoulders, Knees, and Toes is a slightly different spin on the original, with the purpose of gross-motor planning and a lot of silly fun. Start with the group sitting in *Butterfly-Flutterby*. The song cadence might need to be slower than usual to allow enough time to do the poses.

Heads—Hands are on top of the head, elbows bent out to the side.

Shoulders—Fingertips move down to shoulder joint, and elbows move front to back, like a butterfly.

Knees—Knees flap up and down like a butterfly.

Toes—Hands drop to the feet, and the head hangs close to the toes in a forward fold.

Repeat three times.

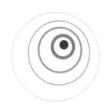

Monkey See, Monkey Do

The purpose of this game is to help children focus their attention. Start out by telling your group that monkeys tend to be very silly and like to copy what they see. Then tell them they are going to be doing the same. Since monkeys can't speak, there will be no talking, and the children will need to rely on their seeing eyes to know what to do. You will be doing poses in sequence for them to copy. If you catch someone not following the directions, you can invite them to sit in *Butterfly-Flutterby* for a turn. Here are some sample pose sequences to try:

> *Hop to It, Mountain, Tall Mountain, Sparkling Star, Satellite, Tall Mountain, Gorilla*
>
> *Butterfly-Flutterby, Smell the Flowers, Table, Hop to It, Ostrich, Gorilla, Downward Dog, Rock*
>
> *Seashell, Sea Star, Peaceful Piggy, Row Your Boat, Sally the Camel, Bug, Crocodile in the Mud*
>
> *Ostrich, Surfer, Teapot, Ostrich, Surfer, Teapot, Ostrich, Tall Mountain, Downward Dog, Rock*

Monkey Toes

Monkey Toes is a lot of fun, and it develops balance, visual acuity, focus, and gross- and fine-motor coordination—quite a lot packaged up as a game! It is best to play this with children ages four and up. Before starting, count out enough marbles for your group size—each child will need about three marbles to retrieve. Have the children remove socks and shoes for this one, and then have them line up to create a "starting line." Explain, "We have a fun and exciting game to play. It involves picking up things, but instead of using our hands, we are going to be using our feet! We are going to be picking up the spilled marbles with our toes and dropping them in the container!" Remind them that this game is not a race but will involve working together to get all of the marbles picked up.

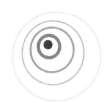

Begin by rolling the precounted marbles (for easy and worry-free retrieval) out into the designated area, which should be big enough for children to move around freely but contained enough so that the marbles are easy to retrieve. A rug is preferable to a smooth surface. Count to three, say "Go," and let the children begin walking around and picking up the marbles and dropping them in the container on the floor. The children will have a great time and become very proud of their skill. (A low, wide container such as a plate or a low basket works best and is the easiest target for the marbles. You may even want to gently hold it so that it won't get knocked over.)

Skidamarinky Dinky Dink, Skidamarinky Do

Have the children stand with their legs apart. Begin singing together, "Skidamarinky dinky dink, skidamarinky do!" As you sing the first line, the children breathe in and move their arms up above their heads, put their hands together, and sway their upper bodies from side to side as they breathe in and out. Then, breathing out, they fold forward with legs still wide and continue swaying back and forth as all sing, "I love you."

For the next "skidamarinky dinky dink, skidamarinky do," breathe the upper bodies back up and slide feet together. With hands over head and fingertips touching to form the moon, sing the last lines: "I love you in the morning and in the afternoon, I love you in the evening underneath the moon." This may sound complicated, but it is adorable, fast, and fun!

We're All Connected

The philosophy of yoga emphasizes union or connection; in fact, the word *yoga* means "union." This game is a powerful and fun way to show how we are all connected, how the action of one affects all, and how we support one another. You will need to purchase a UFO ball, which can often be found at scientific or educational stores, or online. They cost about five dollars. The ball

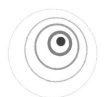

resembles a Ping-Pong ball with two little metal bars on top. When both contacts are touched, the ball lights up and makes a very interesting noise.

Begin by inviting the children to gather in a circle, seated. Instruct them to hold hands. You will be positioned with one of your fingers on the metal contact, and the child (or classroom assistant) next to you should place a finger on the other contact. When everyone is connected, the ball will begin to make its sound. If someone breaks the contact, it stops—like magic! You can instruct different children alternately to break the contact and stop the sound. It becomes a lot of fun. (The ball has a battery in it, and it works by both contacts being touched. Our bodies allow the current to travel through the group until someone breaks it.)

Yoga Bear Says

Yoga Bear Says is the equivalent of Simon Says, where you give directions and the children only follow them when you first say, "Yoga Bear says." The game promotes listening and recall of poses, so you won't want to play it until the children are familiar with or have at least done the poses. Mistakes can have no consequence, or older children can sit "out" in *Butterfly-Flutterby* for a turn, then come back to the game. Here's an example of how the game might go:

> "Yoga Bear says *Hop to It*, Yoga Bear says, 'Stand still.' Oh, I see Emma can rest in *Butterfly-Flutterby*.

> "Yoga Bear says *Ostrich. Yoga Bear says *Satellite. Gorilla*. Oh my goodness, Noah, you can rest in *Butterfly-Flutterby*. Emma, it's time for you to come back."

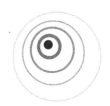

You get the idea! Are you smiling, envisioning this game? One fun thing you can do before starting is have the children gently tug their earlobes. Inform them that they really need their listening ears for this game, and a few gentle pulls will really help them listen.

YOGAMAGINATION

If brain breaks and yoga games are like the warm-up activities of your yoga program, yogamagination is the main event. This is the most similar to what people generally think of as a yoga class—an extended period of poses done in sequence. But because this is a class for young children, it includes more imagination—and it's more fun! Yoga postures, mindful movements, and breathing techniques incorporated into stories you create set the stage to enhance your curriculum in purposeful and playful ways while making the overall classroom experience support physical, cognitive, and social-emotional growth. Pretty amazing, right?

Topics

Your learning objective provides the blueprint for each yogamagination session. Theming and a little bit of planning go a long way to support this fun and valuable experience. Take inventory of your lesson plans and your curriculum units for your idea base. You may be studying the farm, the rain forest, weather, seasons, the tall grass, feelings, family, transportation, shapes and forms, the five senses, the environment, transformation/change, or other areas. Perhaps you are working on body awareness and positional words, self-esteem, manners, emotional balance, or healthy bodies. All of these translate to a yogamagination excursion that supports self-discovery and learning. Or, instead of focusing on a particular subject, you can hold a class to adjust the energy of your group, offering an energizing class on a rainy Monday morning or

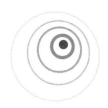

a calming class at the end of a busy day. Self-discovery and learning happen here too! You may also tie in some of the concepts of yoga as part of your class learning intention. These might include the following, many of which are used in our sample lesson plans.

- **Nonharming**—*Treating others, your surroundings, and yourself with respect* (segments that have to do with the natural world).

- **Self-Study**—*Responsible behavior, respecting yourself, knowing yourself* (self-awareness or relating to children's families and others).

- **Something Bigger Than Ourselves**—*Charitable intent, sharing* (cooperation, sharing, dedication).

- **Purity**—*Cleanliness in our environment, body, food, and mind* (environmental study, hygiene and daily habits, healthy eating).

- **Contentment**—*Being happy with things the way they are, being happy with yourself, patience* (learning acceptance and self-acceptance, gratitude and giving thanks).

- **Truth**—*Being true to yourself, being honest, resisting peer pressure* (reinforcement of honesty, integrity, positive self-esteem).

Sequencing

We advise you to begin yogamagination sessions with a breathing activity to unify the group, and then choose poses that support your story theme. A typical sequence starts with seated poses, builds to active and standing poses, and cools down with forward-folding or other calming poses on the belly or back. In some cases, especially if you are following a story, a different sequence of poses may be in order. The only rule you should always follow is

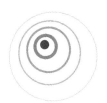

to end with a calming pose. This will often be Rest pose but can also be another quiet, still pose such as Sea Star or Crocodile in the Mud. Keep in mind that it will be easier for children to settle into a resting pose if one or two other calming poses precede it. Remember, forward folds, where the head is released and the chin dropped, draw the body inward and calm the nervous system, as do many poses done on the back or belly. Look back at the notations in chapter 4 for reminders about which poses are calming.

Pacing

It's very common when starting out to talk too quickly. The scripts and stories we offer below may appear to move fast, but successful yogamaginations actually go slowly! Speak at a slow pace, stopping to breathe and pausing in steadiness to demonstrate and do the poses with your eager yoga friends. For poses that move, such as Ostrich, repeat up to three times. Overall, one to two minutes for each pose is a good rule of thumb. Time yourself for a better sense of your own pacing.

TEACHER TIME

In this book, we give you a large toolbox of poses, breaths, and scripts to support your foray into yogamagination and more. But we encourage you to be creative! Change the scripts to suit your style and your children's needs. As you get comfortable, use the tools as stepping-stones to spur your own journeys of the imagination. Invent your own stories. Poses can be adapted; for example, Rock can easily be Egg, Seed, Mouse, or something else you dream up. Invite children to make up their own poses as well. Often some children will say they want to be something not listed as a pose. Don't hesitate to allow your own and your students' creativity to flow—it makes yoga that much more fun!

Sample Lesson Plans for Yogamagination with a Gross-Motor Focus

Following are some sample classes where the primary goal is gross-motor development. While some of the later yogamagination plans are more elaborate, the scripts for energy, strength, and so on are not written in as much detail because the purpose is very focused here. These plans will take less time as well. The length may be appropriate for younger groups and groups just starting out with yoga. Later these plans might ultimately be plugged into your day like a long brain break or perhaps used with a small group during free play. You might choose to use them with specific students who need some help in developing certain skills, such as core strength, or with everyone. Note that yogamagination plans are written in narrative form, as a teacher might speak. Use these as a starting point and adapt as much as you like. When you see a pose in *italic*, stop to do that pose with your group. (Sometimes the pose name differs slightly from the name in chapter 4 to make it fit the story. You'll be able to understand which pose is meant.)

Balance

"Friends, our balance is important and helps us do all sorts of things. Today it might be fun to do some yoga poses that help us get better at balance. And it might be an exciting adventure for us! I bet that if we keep trying these poses over time, our balance is going to get even better. Let's begin. Stand strong and straight like a *Mountain*. And now let's *Go for a Walk* up the mountain. At the tippy top I see a big *Tree* standing straight and so tall that it touches the sky with its branches while its roots go down deep. That's how it stays steady on the side of the *Mountain*. If you look hard, you may see a *Flying Bird* in that tree. The bird takes off into the sky and flies up like an *Airplane*! Your balancing is great, friends! Let's take a rest in *Rock* pose."

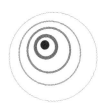

Body Awareness/Proprioception

"We are going to hike to a *Mountain* today! Come onto your backs, friends, and if it feels okay, close your eyes and feel the ground under you. Wait a minute—let's *Catch a Ball* that's rolling away. Let's follow it! Notice how your back feels on the floor. The ball takes us to a *Bridge*, and we cross over it. We've crossed the *Bridge*, and I see the *Mountain*. It is standing still and steady on the earth. Maybe you can feel strong and steady too. It looks very cold there; I think I see snow on top. Better put on our *Coat Sleeves* to stay warm on our hike. Let's *Go for a Walk* up the mountain! Whew, let's stand under this *Tree* and take a break. Oh my goodness, look over there—there is a *Downward Dog*! What is he doing here? Do you think he is looking for his ball? Let's see if it's behind that *Rock*."

Calming 1

"My friends, I think it is time for some yoga. It has been a busy morning, and we might feel a little better after doing some yoga. Let's all sit down in *Easy Peasy*. I invite you to close your eyes if that feels good for you and imagine green *Trees* and bushes, and a warm breeze. We are going to a pretend mountainside in Africa. Let's take three big breaths together and listen to the sounds around us. Do you hear the *Trees* and bushes moving in the wind? Aah. Let's open our eyes and look around. Beautiful *Butterflies* are everywhere, landing right near us. Let's get on our *Hands and Knees* to watch them. Wow, beautiful! [Ask the children to say quietly what colors they see.] I see friendly *Downward Dogs*, and now I hear something walking this way—listen. There is a family of *Gorillas* coming to see us! Let's *Take a Walk* so we don't disturb them. We keep walking until we come to the top of the *Mountain*, and we are very still. Let's take three big breaths while we are here. All around are green *Trees* and more *Gorillas*. Right nearby there is a stream, and in it there are some *Crocodiles* sleeping. We curl up beside a *Rock* and have a *Rest*."

Calming 2

"It's group time; let's all come together. Some things can make me feel really happy. What makes you happy? [If your group is small enough, you can let the children all share one thing.] Maybe it's someone you love, or maybe you need a little love. Let's practice our *Happy Heart* breathing. [This guided meditation takes a little time, so there are fewer poses in this yoga session.] Now open your eyes, take a giant breath in, and then let it out of your mouth with a sound. Great job! You know what might be nice? A picnic by the lake. I see *Butterflies Fluttering* by; they make me feel happy in my heart! There are happy *Cows* eating grass nearby, and maybe you hear the sound of the water nearby and notice it is just like your breath, moving in and out like waves [*Ocean Breath*].

"I see a *Kitty* sitting in the sun on a *Rock*. I would like my dog to come, and she bows like a *Downward Dog* because she is happy too! I'm hungry, and I think we should think about our snack. Let's go sit on that *Rock* so we can see the lake and make a *Sandwich*. That was nice! Look over there—some *Seashells* are around the edge of the lake. They are really pretty. And I am so happy. Let's lie on our backs and pretend we are *Sea Stars*. Feel your belly go up and down like the waves in the lake."

Energy 1

"Good morning, friends! I see everyone looking a little sleepy today—me too! Let's get our energy moving with some yoga time! It's such a gray day today; let's take a quick pretend trip to the zoo to visit a few animal friends. We don't have very long, so we might want to hurry. Let's *Run* to get there. Come down on *Hands and Knees* so we can visit the children's section and see the *Cows and Kitties* and *Downward Dogs*. Here at the zoo, feel the *Warmth of the Sun* shining down! I see *Ostriches*, and they lift their heads up and down. Let's come down to our *Hands and Knees* again so we can watch. Look over there—it's *Sally the Camel*, and she is going to give us a ride! Whew, that was fun! Let's go look over there—it's

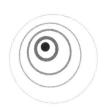

the *Gorillas Tapping* their chests. Maybe we should go sit on a *Rock* and watch the slithery *Snake*. Wow, this has been a fun trip. I'm ready to go back to the *Rock*, and then maybe take a short *Rest*."

Energy 2

"Oh my goodness, I see a bunny, and he is twitching his nose and breathing hard. I think he wants us to follow him! Let's try to breathe like the bunny [*Bunny Breath*]. Wait, there he goes. We had better *Hop to It* after him! Oh my goodness, he took us to where it is *Raining*—it is kind of fun to get wet! And just like that, it stops, and look at that, a beautiful *Rainbow*. This is a magical place we have followed that bunny to. I see a *Sparkling Star*, and over there is the *Moon*. I think maybe we have come to Nursery Rhyme Land. Let's come down to our *Hands and Knees* so we can get on that *Rocking Horse* and ride. It turns into a *Rock*! Come over to your backs, and let's go over *London Bridge*. Then we curl up in a magic *Seashell*, and it rocks and rolls us home to *Rest*."

Gross Motor 1

"Did you ever want to go on an adventure to the ocean? Let's go—we will be safe and have fun together! Let's begin by *Riding Our Bikes* to the dock. We pedal up the hills and down the hills until we get there. Whew, we made it! Look, there is our *Boat*. It is a little windy out, and the *Boat* rocks a little, but we are having fun! The waves calm down just in time for us to see a gigantic sea *Turtle* swimming beside us. Then we look on the other side, and there is a beautiful *Shark* swimming by peacefully—wow! There are so many living things in the sea. It is time to go back! Our *Boat* takes us to the dock so we can *Ride Our Bikes* back here, but guess what? A *Sea Star* came back with us! Let's lie on our backs and imagine we are one while we *Rest*."

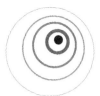

Gross Motor 2

"What a beautiful day it is! It might be fun to explore a meadow—a big field full of flowers, grass, and the animals that live there. Let's *Go for a Walk* and explore it! My goodness, the grass [rubbing palms together to make the sound] is so very tall that it is making it a little harder to walk. Pick your feet up high! Perhaps we should use our giant *Scissors* to trim it down a little to make our exploring easier. Our breathing sounds like the *Scissors* cutting grass! Whew, that is better. Now I can see a bunch of frogs—*Hop to It*! And I see some baby *Horses* kicking up their feet while they explore the meadow. Maybe we should go sit under the *Tree* and watch some more. Do you see something moving over there? It's a slithering *Snake*. Now it's going under that *Rock*!"

Strength 1

"It's time for us to do the Dino . . . *Dino Breath*! Dinosaurs were mostly very strong and powerful. Today we are going to do some yoga time poses that will help us feel strong too!

"Now, I am going to see if we can all stand big, still, and strong like a *Mountain.* Let's take five breaths here together. That was great, friends. Fold over and be a *Gorilla*; you might notice your belly muscles when we lift up. Stand with your feet wide and bring your hands together like mine, and after we breathe our arms up, we are going to reach our arms down and say, 'Hah.' Let's be strong like a *Wood Chopper* [repeat two more times]. Whew, you guys are doing great! Can you fly high like a *Flying Bird*? Keep your wings strong. What about kicking like a *Horse*? Come to *Downward Dog* and, being very careful just like me, kick. Now kick three times. That is fantastic! I feel stronger already just watching you, friends. Let's take a break and *Gorilla* hang for a few breaths. Breathe back up to *Mountain*, and let's stay here for a few breaths, very still and strong. You might even notice your heart is beating a little stronger. Now come rest in *Rock* pose. Turn over onto your backs, and breathe your arms and legs straight up. Now move

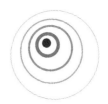

them just like me and be a *Sloth*; you might feel this in your belly muscles too! Now, after all our good work, let's be *Peaceful Piggies* and pretend we are rolling in the mud to cool us. Aah—let's *Rest* right here."

Strength 2

"Come to yoga time, sit down in *Easy Peasy*, and get ready for a trip to the beach. We are going to have a great time. Let's *Go for a Walk* and feel the *Warmth of the Sun*. Let's *Catch a Ball* here on the beach. Wow, I feel warmer! Now let's go *Surfing*—here comes the wave. Whew! Drop down on your tummy. Here comes another wave. Push up to *Downward Dog*, and let's stand up to *Surf* this one. Wow, that was really hard work! Come down onto your bellies, friends. There are *Silly Seals* on the beach, and they are clapping for us! Let's be like them. They go rest on the *Rocks*, and we go cool off on the *Slippy Slide*. Now it is time for a *Boat* ride. We gather *Seashells* in a net and some *Sea Stars* too. Let's all *Rest* like a sea star and feel the waves carry us home."

Using the Plans as a Workbook Form

Now is the time for you to review this grouping of plans and think about how to make them your own. Looking at these sequences, ask yourself how you would string them together in your voice. Based on the cueing given, how would you prompt your class? Perhaps you might add or remove some things based on your children and their individual needs.

To help you think about this and plan future classes, we're including some of the lesson plans presented above in chart form. This provides an easier reference and also a template you can use for your own planning. Two additional lesson plans are included here that were not presented above. They are designed to support all-around gross-motor development. How would you develop these into a full class for your group?

Focus	Breath	Warm-Up	Active	Cooldown
Energy 1	Running	Hands and Knees Cow/Kitty Downward Dog	Warmth of the Sun Ostrich Hands and Knees Sally the Camel Gorilla Tapping	Rock Snake Rock Rest
Energy 2	Bunny	Hop to It Let It Rain	Who Can Make a Rainbow? Sparkling Star Moon in the Sky Hands and Knees Rocking Horse	Rock London Bridge Seashell Rest
Calming 1	Ocean (The targeted breath is at the end on this one.)	Easy Peasy Butterfly-Flutterby Hands and Knees Downward Dog	Gorilla Go for a Walk Mountain Tree Gorilla	Crocodile in the Mud Rock Rest
Calming 2	Happy Heart Ocean	Butterfly-Flutterby Kitty	Rock Downward Dog Rock Sandwich	Seashell Sea Star
Strength 1	Dino	Mountain Gorilla	Wood Chopper Flying Bird Horse Gorilla Mountain Rock	Sloth Peaceful Piggy Rest
Strength 2	Sun (The targeted breath is in the middle of this one.)	Easy Peasy Go for a Walk Warmth of the Sun	Surfer Downward Dog Silly Seal Rock Slippy Slide	Row Your Boat Seashell Sea Star Rest
All-Around 1	Buzzing	Easy Peasy Wheels on the Bus	Cow/Kitty Downward Dog Mountain Tree Teapot	Peaceful Piggy Rest
All-Around 2	Snakey	Rock Snake Rock	Downward Dog Go for a Walk Mountain Warrior Gorilla Lion	Rock Rest

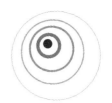

Planning a Yogamagination Based on Curriculum

This section is going to walk you through planning a yogamagination that will enhance your curriculum. When young children act out a concept or story through movement, they understand it in a kinesthetic way. Yoga poses allow children to feel the lessons in their bodies, creating deeper understanding. For some children, this is their primary way of absorbing new information. For others, learning through movement adds a new level of comprehension. This is true whether the lesson is about science, stories, or social-emotional topics like self-esteem.

Yoga poses are ideal for kinesthetic learning. Take a look at this list of poses and see if you can sense a curriculum topic: *Easy Peasy*, *Butterfly-Flutterby*, *Hop to It*, *Feel the Breeze*, *Tree*, *Flying Bird*, *Go for a Walk*, *Mountain*, *Smell the Flowers*, *Rock*, and *Rest*. Reading through this sequence of poses, did you guess that this yogamagination supports learning about spring? If so, you would be correct!

Just by connecting the movement of the poses with their names, you offer your group a kinesthetic learning experience. Weaving the poses into a narrative makes it a cognitive experience as well, supporting true all-around learning. Following is one example of a way to tie the poses together into a story about a spring walk. This would be best suited to do in the spring so children have direct experience with the topic you are teaching.

"Today, my friends, we are going to take a yogamagination spring walk. Many changes take place in the spring. Nature gives us so many things to see, smell, hear, and touch. Let's go on an adventure! What do you think you might see on our spring walk? [Invite comments.] Okay, let's find out!

"Come and let's sit in *Easy Peasy* pose. I invite you to close your eyes if that feels okay to you. Imagine that it is a beautiful day like today and the season is spring. The air is just starting to warm up, and you don't even have to wear a jacket! I think I smell something special and hear something calling us to explore. Open your

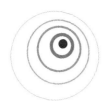

eyes. I see a *Butterfly-Flutterby*! I see so many colors. Look over at the puddle from all the spring *Rain*—there's a frog *Hopping to It*! [Stand.] Take a big breath in and lift your arms up and *Feel the Breeze* blow. It feels so good! And it is making the tiny green leaves on the *Tree* move gently. Remember in winter when the trees had no leaves? Wait, I hear something—it's a *Stork*! That's a kind of bird. Let's sing like a bird; take a big breath in and sing. Tweet! Now let's *Go for a Walk* up the *Mountain*. Wow, that was a little bit of work! I am feeling a little warm. Let's sit down in this beautiful grass and *Smell the Flowers*. We are all going to sit down on a *Rock*. And now, let's move into *Rest*."

Take a moment to reflect on the script. Can you hear yourself doing it? What parts would you use, and what would you change? Take a deep breath yourself, and practice leading the walk aloud. Find a suitable place and practice again, adding in the poses. Remember to speak slowly and leave plenty of time for long, slow breaths. Let your creativity flow so the story becomes *your* story.

Consider what other discoveries and happenings you might include in yogamaginations to help children learn about spring.

BRINGING THE NATURAL WORLD INTO PLAY

Yoga brings both science and the natural world to life, so embrace this opportunity in your classroom! It can vastly enrich your curriculum. For many children, the outdoor world is something they may see only on a screen. Lessons on nature can bring the experience into their bodies through poses such as *Stormy Weather, Warmth of the Sun, Who Can Make a Rainbow?*, and many others. Integrate your yoga nature lessons with real outdoor experiences whenever possible. For example, you could have the children find a tree to watch during the seasons to allow them to observe change. Let them show you how their tree looks in *Tree* pose. The sky is the limit, and it is a very real way to integrate science and nature into your lessons.

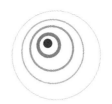

You could come back to this journey repeatedly over a period of time, one day looking at baby animals, another day creating a plan around the life cycle of the frog or butterfly. To make it a yogamagination journey, just be sure to include yoga movement with each turn of the story. You might also include a discussion of acceptance of change, which relates to the yoga concept of contentment. Growth means change, which is sometimes welcome but sometimes less so. For example, tadpoles learn to accept their new selves. How might this relate to what your children are experiencing?

Sample Lesson Plans for Yogamagination with a Curriculum, Science, or Yoga Focus

Below are some sample lesson plans for you to use. Each is built around a curriculum theme from science or social-emotional learning, along with a related yoga concept. These plans are presented in a fuller format than the gross-motor plans, including setting the stage activities and story extensions before and after the narrative. The purpose is to encourage full, deep learning. As always, use the plans as offered or as stepping-stones to creating your own yogamagination journeys.

Down on the Farm (Healthy Eating/Connecting to the Food Source)

Yoga concept: Patience or purity

Setting the stage: Some fruits and vegetables, mini hay bale, seed packs, pictures of farm silos, crops, tractors.

Discuss: "What happens on a farm? What lives there? Grows there? What might happen if there were no farms?"

Poses: Ride My Bike, Warmth of the Sun, Tree, Wood Chopper (Ostrich/Elephant), Horse, Cow, Kitty, Downward Dog, Rock, Rest

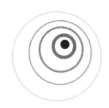

Narrative: "We are going to *Ride Our Bikes* to the farm. Let's put on our helmets. [Place hands behind head, turn right, turn left.] Okay, let's pedal slowly, going uphill. Whew, pedal fast as we roll downhill. [Do this twice more.] The *Warmth of the Sun* is shining on us and helping grow the food. I see apple *Trees* with shiny red apples. [Children can make their hands into fists to be apples.] The farmer is in the field, chopping hay [*Wood Chopper*]. He is going to use this hay to feed the *Horse* and *Cow* on the farm. Do you hear the cow moo? On the fence there is a *Kitty*, and sitting by him is the farm *Dog*. Over by the dog is a *Rock*. Let's go sit down, cool off, and take a *Rest* here."

Story extension: Read *The Carrot Seed* by Ruth Krauss. Discuss what goes into growing vegetables and fruit. Ask, "How does the sun help? The rain? What did it take for the carrot seed to grow?"

I Like Me (Positive Self-Image)

Yoga concept: Self-study

Setting the stage: Have the children bring in baby pictures and one or two more photos where they are progressively older. Have mirrors for them to look at themselves. If space and time allow, you can create a bulletin board called "I Like Me," writing what the children say they like about themselves under their photos.

Discuss: "What do you like about yourself? What can you do now that you couldn't when you were smaller? How does that make you feel?"

Poses: This is a more open-ended lesson plan, so you can choose the poses depending on your group's needs that particular day. Back-bending poses energize and create a sense of fearlessness, so choose a few of these to create a positive lift!

1. *Cow/Kitty, Sally the Camel, Table, London Bridge, Shark, Rock, Rest*

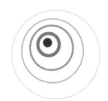

2. Poses that allow children to feel strong and empowered, allowing them to demonstrate their gross-motor development and balancing skills. Here are some possibilities: *Slippy Slide*, *Hop to It*, *Mountain*, *L on the Wall*, *Warrior*, *Airplane*, *Tall Mountain*, *Rocking Horse*, *Rock*.

Story extension: Read *My Many Colored Days* by Dr. Seuss. (You can also create another yogamagination journey doing poses that mirror the book.) Ask the children what color they feel like when they are happy, sad, and so on. Another story option is *The Story of Ferdinand* by Munro Leaf. Discuss how Ferdinand was different. Ask, "What makes you different? The same? Is it okay to be different?"

Let's All Come Together (Teamwork and Cooperation)

Yoga concept: Something bigger than ourselves.

Setting the stage: Pictures of groups of people working, playing, or eating together (make them as diverse as you can), a globe, things from different countries. This can turn into a lot of educational fun. You might even have a multicultural food day.

Discuss: "How should we treat others? How do you like to be treated? How can we take care of others and their feelings?"

Poses: Seesaw, *Rope Pull*, *Standing House*, *Double W*, *We're All Connected*

Narrative: Choose a partner for each child, and switch the partners on different days. Try to choose partners about the same size. Explain to them that we need to remember to treat our partners like we want them to treat us. If there is too much silliness, you may have to stop or switch partners. Children especially enjoy doing these poses, and the circle at the end is a much asked for activity.

Story extension: Read *Seven Blind Mice* by Ed Young. Discuss how the mice struggle to work together, each one just doing one part—this story is great for teaching how to see the whole and what could happen if we come together! Invite the children to try coming together with a friend or family member.

The Rain Forest (Environmental Awareness)

Yoga concept: Purity or nonharming, patience

Setting the stage: Bromeliads, tropical flowers, bright feathers, pictures of the habitat and its inhabitants, a globe, rain stick.

Discuss: "Why is it called a rain forest? What is a habitat?"

Poses for Lesson 1: Airplane, *Warmth of the Sun*, Airplane [other side], *Tree, Forest, Hop to It, Stork, Snake, Rock, Sloth, Rest*

Narrative: "Today our yogamagination is taking us far away to a special place where it is very warm and rainy. It is called the rain forest. We need to take care of the rain forest because the animals that live there can't live anywhere else. We will be visiting them over the next few days.

"We will need to travel by *Airplane*. The plane is taking off; feel the *Warmth of the Sun* [breathe arms up]. Now it is time for the *Airplane* to land. [Do *Airplane* raising the opposite leg.] We land in the middle of a big group of *Trees*. They create the *Forest* that took a very long time to grow. In the trees we hear and see monkeys *Hop to It*, and we see a colorful big bird [*Stork*] and see it fly! I hear something—look, it is a slithering *Snake*, and he curls up by a *Rock*. Oh my, I see a very special animal, my favorite, in the trees over our heads—it is a *Sloth*. He is slow and patient. Now, let's *Rest* right here under the trees."

Story extension: Read *"Slowly, Slowly, Slowly," Said the Sloth* by Eric Carle. Discuss how hard it is to be patient. Ask, "What does it mean to be patient? What are times when you feel upset because you have to wait?"

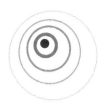

Poses for Lesson 2: *Forest, Easy Peasy, Smell the Flowers, Warmth of the Sun, Stormy Weather, Warmth of the Sun* [repeat], *Who Can Make a Rainbow?, Row Your Boat, Bug, Crocodile in the Mud, Rest*

Narrative: "Let's explore the *Rain Forest* more today—there is much to see and discover! As we sit here [*Easy Peasy*], I *Smell Flowers* of all kinds. Do you? How do they smell? I feel the *Warm Sun* helping them grow. Wait, do you hear something? It's thunder and lightning, but it isn't frightening. All of a sudden, it starts to *Storm*. It storms slow, and then fast, and then slows down and stops. I feel the *Warmth of the Sun* again. Whew, look, there is something in the sky—a *Rainbow*! I see a river by its end. Let's *Row Our Boats* there. There are lots of *Bugs* around, and I see *Crocodiles in the Mud*. Let's stop here and *Rest*."

Story extension: Read *Verdi* by Janell Cannon.

Transformation Station (Change)

Yoga concept: Contentment

Setting the stage: If possible, have seeds and the plant or vegetable they turn into, pictures of life cycles of chicks, frogs, or butterflies, pictures of a tree in each season. This is a great activity to do when you have the ability to perhaps get a butterfly garden or chick hatching project.

Discuss: "Everything changes. What are some things you notice changing every day?" Pick a tree near your classroom that you can observe daily and record the changes.

Poses: Do these poses in a series as they are grouped below. Flow from one to another to act out the transformation.

Mountain, Mountain [repeat], L on the Wall, Rock

Wiggly Worm, Smell the Flowers, Caterpillar Cocoon, Butterfly-Flutterby

Cow/Kitty, Downward Dog, Rock [repeat]

Rock, Wiggly Worm, Bug, Hop to It

Story extension: Read *Miss Maple's Seeds* by Eliza Wheeler. Discuss how plants grow and seasons change. Ask, "Do you like it when things change? How does it make you feel? Sometimes changes are a lot better than we thought they would be!"

Trip to the Zoo (Environmental Awareness, Respect for Others)

Yoga concept: Nonharming

Setting the stage: Puzzles, games, and other activities involving animals you see in a zoo.

Discuss: "Have you visited a zoo? Would you like to? What animals might you see?"

Poses: *Wheels on the Bus, Turtle, Sally the Camel, Elephant (Wood Chopper/Ostrich), Gorilla, Gorilla Tapping, Lion, Snake, Crocodile in the Mud, Wheels on the Bus* [repeat]

Narrative: "Friends, today we're going to take an imaginary trip to the zoo! We're going to ride a *Bus* to get there. Let's start out slowly as we leave school. Now we can go faster! Okay, slow down again; here we are at the zoo! The first animals we see are *Turtles*. Turtles are slow, quiet animals, so let's be quiet so we don't disturb them. See how they hide inside their shells? Let's do that too. Now we come to a camel. Do you think her name is *Sally the Camel*? Put your hands on your hump! Next is an *Elephant*. She must be hot, because she's spraying water over her back. Now I see a big *Gorilla*! Look, he's *Tapping* his chest. The *Lion* cage is next. Let's listen to the lions roar. Now lie on your belly. What animal do you think we're going to see next that slithers on its belly? That's right, a *Snake*! There is a river in the zoo. There's a *Crocodile*, resting in the sun. Let's *Rest* like the crocodile. Roll onto your back. Pretend you have a blanket and we're resting in the cool shade at the zoo.

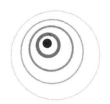

[Wait.] Now to end, we're going to take a nice, slow ride home on the *Bus*. We're going very slowly because we already rested. Here we are, back at school!"

Story extension: Read *Giraffes Can't Dance* by Giles Andreae. Invite the children to dance like their favorite animal.

ACT OUT A STORY

Everybody, young and old, loves a good story! You can use that love for literature to enhance your curriculum. Stories can teach us about patience or strength of character, and they can connect us to our own emotions. All of these lessons can expand your classroom activities around social-emotional learning. Acting out a story through yoga is a great way to enhance the learning experience and bring it to life for your children.

Coordinating your curriculum units with poems and stories draws children in and piques their interest. Moving and acting out stories creates body memory, and by acting out a story, the children will become part of it. They may go home and reenact it again and again.

When choosing a story to use, be sure you can integrate yoga poses and that the story is short enough to hold the children's attention. This is where you may need to think on your feet a little and adapt existing postures to fit the story. Most of all, acting out a story inspires creativity on both your parts. You can read the story and then act it out with your children and do the poses together. If you and your group have been doing yogamagination journeys for a while, an option is to have the children do the poses while you are reading the story out loud. You can also invite them to make up poses for story features that don't already have one.

Let's look at some books that lend themselves nicely to this activity. Remember, this list is only a starting point. Many other books would be quite appropriate—probably including some that are already on your bookshelf! Sample books are given below with suggestions for poses you can use.

Little Cloud by Eric Carle (Philomel Books, 1996). *Standing House, Kitty* (for sheep), *Airplane, Shark, Tree,* and *Bunny, Hop to It, Sparkling Star, Stormy Weather,* and *Let It Rain.*

Giraffes Can't Dance by Giles Andreae (Scholastic, 1999). *Giraffe* (breathing the arms up and hands coming together over head), *Go for a Walk, Lion, Ostrich, Hop to It, Horse* (for zebra), *Mountain, Moon in the Sky, Feel the Breeze,* freeform movement. Use this book as an opportunity to talk about treating others kindly and being an individual.

The Mitten by Jan Brett (G. P. Putnam's Sons, 1989). Rubbing the hands and placing them on the face (warm mittens), *Hop to It, Flying Bird, Kitty* (for hedgehog), *Downward Dog, Rock* (as mouse), coming onto their backs, pulling their knees to the belly, and exploding like the mitten by opening arms and legs out as you would for *Caterpillar Cocoon.*

Miss Maple's Seeds by Eliza Wheeler (Puffin Books, 2017). *Stork, Rock* (as seed), rubbing the hands, *Hop to It, Feel the Breeze,* rubbing hands (repeat), touch the sky and reach your toes for snow, *Stormy Weather, Feel the Breeze, Rock* (as seed), *Tree, Teapot, Row Your Boat* (as a rocker), *Rock, Rest.*

Sometimes I Like to Curl Up in a Ball by Vicki Churchill (Sterling, 2001). *Rock, Butterfly-Flutterby, Hop to It, Lion, Go for a Walk,* running breath, *Tree, Turtle, Rock.*

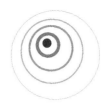

Here are more suggestions that both you and your children will find delightful. Some of them lend themselves to acting out each page with movement. Some of them explore yoga concepts and may be more suited for sitting and listening to most of the pages, with just a few movements to help keep children interested and to integrate the concepts. Read and choose what will work best with your group.

Seven Blind Mice by Ed Young (Philomel Books, 1992)

The Carrot Seed by Ruth Krauss (Scholastic, 1945)

Twinkle, Twinkle, Little Star by Iza Trapani (Charlesbridge, 1997)

While I Sleep by Mary Calhoun (William Morrow & Co., 1992)

The Empty Pot by Demi (Square Fish, 1996)

My Many Colored Days by Dr. Seuss (Alfred A. Knopf, 1996)

Ahn's Anger by Gail Silver (Plum Blossom Books, 2009)

Visiting Feelings by Lauren Rubenstein (Magination Press, 2014)

GUIDED IMAGERY

Think of a time when you've felt profoundly good inside, perhaps in front of a cozy fire or while watching a sunset at the beach. The happiness reaches your bones, and it seems like everything is right with the world, if only for that one brief moment. Children enjoy these feelings too. Using guided imagery, you can create experiences for them that have the power to evoke those calm, peaceful feelings. Guided imagery gives children a break from all the stimulation going on around them and shifts their attention inward. It makes an excellent start to naptime. When you offer these activities, you give the children a chance to slow down and tune in to their internal world. In addition, these sessions provide a great way to exercise the muscles that power their imaginations.

GUIDED IMAGERY AND FEELINGS

Note that peace and happiness are not the only emotions that might arise during guided imagery exercises. Having quiet, internal experiences may release less comfortable feelings, including fear and anger. Weave words of reassurance and safety through your meditation, and then give children a way to express whatever feelings they had once the guided meditation is done. For example, invite them to paint or draw their feelings. What colors do they choose? What kinds of motions do they use to make their painting or drawing? If possible, ask each child to tell you about what they are drawing, and with their permission, write their words down on their art. Self-portraits are a lovely way to allow your children to show how they feel. Provide very young children with a silhouette on legal-size paper; older children can attempt to draw their own. Invite them to draw themselves during the guided meditation. Or if they prefer, they could draw something else that makes them feel really good or something else they like about themselves.

Dancing to music is another option. Suggest that children try to listen with their bodies and "speak" their feelings with movements, expressing themselves freely. Take a moment to remind them about safety rules and that any kind of movement is permissible as long as those rules are followed. Classical music with varied tempos works nicely here, such as Vivaldi's *The Four Seasons* or *The Nutcracker* by Tchaikovsky.

There are many ways to bring guided imagery into your classroom. The most important thing is to set the stage. You can choose to do these activities either sitting up or lying down. Be aware of student placement. When next to one another, some children can't help themselves from talking and laughing. Use yourself as a buffer if need be. If you can, and you think it will be okay for the children in your room, turn off some or all of the overhead lights. Fluorescent lighting can be stimulating, and when your room gets quiet enough, you can actually hear the

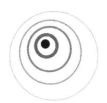

lights hum. To prepare your group for this new and special activity, explain to them that they are going to be using their minds to take them to a special place. With the children in position and the room calm, you can begin. Expect some initial restlessness if this is a new activity, but after a short time, children usually settle in nicely to the imaginary world. If your meditation takes the children on a journey, be sure to always guide them safely back.

Here are a few examples of instructions you can give to guide your children through these calming, imaginative explorations. Speak slowly in a calm, soothing voice.

Ocean

Tell the children, "As you lie on your back, put your hands on your belly. Breathe in and out through your nose. After every breath in, the next out breath will make you feel calmer, warmer, and softer. Feel how when you breathe in, your belly lifts up. [Pause.] And when you breathe out, it lowers back down. [Pause.] The movement is just like the waves in the ocean. Your breath flows in and out without your having to do anything except notice it. As you continue to breathe in and out through your nose, imagine that you are floating on a big, strong raft that keeps you perfectly safe while you ride up and down on the ocean of your breath." Extend this narrative as you choose. For example, you can talk about feeling the warm sun on their bellies, hearing the seagulls, and smelling the salt air. When you're ready to end the exercise, say, "Now it's time for us to leave the ocean. Take a gigantic breath into your belly and breathe out of your mouth. Then pull your knees into your tummy, wrap your arms around your knees, and rock from side to side. Roll onto your side. Give yourself a big hug, and sit up crisscross applesauce."

Magic Carpet

Begin by saying, "Draw an imaginary box around yourself on the
floor. [Demonstrate.] This is your magic carpet. It can take you
anywhere in the world you want to go. Our breath is what's going
to give it the magic power to rise up into the sky. Close your eyes
if you want to, but it's okay if you don't. Breathe slowly and deeply
into your belly. Feel the air in your belly and imagine that it is
lifting your magic carpet up. Remember that your magic carpet
will always keep you safe. Maybe it's going to travel to the house
of someone you love. Maybe it's going to a safari far away, where
you can look down and see wild animals. Maybe it's going to the
moon! Or maybe it's on the way to your very own warm, snug
bed or comfy couch. While you breathe, ride your carpet to the
place you choose. Now I'm going to be quiet for a little bit so you
can stay still and imagine." Pause one to two minutes and let the
children stay with the imagery in their heads. Judge the timing
by their stillness. When they start to get restless, or just before,
it's time to bring them back. Say, "Now it's time to return to our
classroom. Continue breathing in and breathing out. Ride your
magic carpet away from your special place and back here to our
classroom. Let it land slowly and gently on the rug. Take a big
breath into your tummy. This time let it out of your mouth with
a sigh. Pull your knees into your tummy, wrap your arms around
them, and give your body a big hug. Then roll over onto your side.
Take a breath or two. And then come back up to sitting crisscross
applesauce."

Happy Heart

Instruct the children to sit crisscross applesauce, with their eyes
closed if they are willing. Tell them to place their hands, palms
down, on their hearts. Then say, "Take a big breath in through your
nose. Feel your heart lift up. Every time you breathe in, feel your

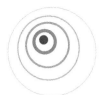

heart fill up with love and peace. Maybe you can imagine it lighting up with a color. Maybe it even gets brighter every time you take a breath. While you breathe, think of a part of you that might need some love right now. And as you breathe into your heart, send your love to that part of you that needs it most. Maybe it's your knee. Maybe it's your tummy. Maybe it's somewhere else. Perhaps your heart needs a little extra love today, especially if you're feeling sad or mad. Perhaps your mind needs some extra love if you are thinking sad or angry thoughts. Send your loving breath wherever it needs to go. As you continue to send love where you need it the most, begin thinking about somebody else—maybe a friend or someone in your family, someone you know who needs your love, or maybe even a pet. Imagine that person. Breathe in, and when you breathe out, let the out breath send that person a big, happy hug. Imagine that person can feel it and is now smiling. Then maybe he or she sends you a hug back. Next time you breathe out, notice how you feel in your body. Sit for a moment with that feeling. Open your eyes if they are closed. Use your arms to give yourself a big, happy hug."

I Can Do Anything

Tell the children that this is a meditation to help them do anything. Introduce it by saying something like this: "Sometimes there are things that are hard for all of us to do. It might be learning something new like riding a bike, zipping your coat, catching a ball, writing your name, or maybe even sharing with someone new. But if you can imagine yourself doing that hard thing, it can help you learn how to do it! Sports players do this. Professional basketball players imagine themselves shooting the ball and getting a basket before they actually throw it. You can do this too. Let's close our eyes, if that feels okay to you. Think about something that you have a hard time doing. Now see yourself in your mind, and see yourself doing that thing—and doing a really good job. Do it again and again in your mind, until you feel like, 'I got this!' Feel how good that feels in your body, in your heart, and in your mind. Remember that feeling. Carry it with you today." Instruct the children to open their eyes. If you want to, you can end with an affirmation. Invite the children to say, "I am strong. I am wonderful. I can do anything." Let them know that anytime they have a hard time doing something, they can try this exercise—it really helps! They may not be able to do their difficult thing perfectly the first time, but they will keep getting better at it.

Peaceful Paws

Have the children bring their "peaceful paws" (hands) together in front of their hearts. Invite them to close their eyes and begin to rub their palms together, creating warmth, love, and peace. They will feel a warm sensation in their palms. Ask them to place one hand on their hearts and one on their bellies and feel that peace, love, and warmth spread inside. Perhaps they can even imagine the peace and love going to someone they know who really needs it, such as their friend or parent.

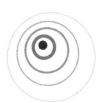

The Rainbow

The Rainbow is what is known as a "body scan," and it can allow children to notice where there is tension in their bodies and how they feel in this moment. This exercise can take some time for adults, but for this age, complete this exercise in perhaps three minutes, no more than five minutes for older preschoolers.

Start by inviting the children to lie down on their backs and close their eyes if they feel comfortable doing so. Tell them, "Imagine a very small rainbow and notice the colors. You don't have to do anything right now but imagine that little rainbow. It shines on your forehead, and you notice how it feels there. Maybe it feels warm, or maybe cool. Or one color is very bright to you. Just notice how that is. [Pause.] The rainbow moves to your shoulder, and you feel it there, and how it is. [Pause.]

"Now your attention follows the rainbow to your other shoulder. Maybe it feels different. [Pause.] The rainbow then moves its light to your leg, and you see how that feels. [Pause.] Notice if it feels warm, cool, light, or heavy as it then moves to your other leg. [Pause.] Just see the beautiful colors of your rainbow as they are. The rainbow travels to your belly, and you feel it there, noticing how it is the same or different. [Pause.] And then your rainbow shines on your heart. Maybe you notice one color more, or how it feels to have the rainbow shine on your heart. Watch and just breathe. And then that rainbow floats up in the sky, and you take a big breath into your tummy and notice how it feels just to lie here. [Pause.] Roll over to your side. [Pause.] And, slowly, come up to sitting in *Easy Peasy*."

Superspecial Senses

The purpose of Superspecial Senses is for your children to learn to distinguish through observation and take their attention to a more refined focus. This meditation can be very helpful if you happen to

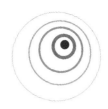

be doing a unit on the senses. You can do just one sense at a time so that the lessons can be extended, or with older preschoolers, you may want to fly high and do them all at once.

Tell your children that you are going to be turning into Super-Sense Heroes so they can notice things that most people might not. That is a pretty special power for sure! Have them sit in *Easy Peasy*, and give the suggestion to close their eyes. Tell them that they are going to be using their super sense of hearing. (Note that this hearing activity on its own makes a great brain break during transition times.)

Begin by saying, "Let your hearing super sense discover what sounds you hear around you. Perhaps you notice the sound of the heater blowing. Perhaps you hear the sound of cars outside or an airplane flying by. Just listen to the layers of all the sounds. Maybe you hear your friend moving or even hear them breathing. [Pause.] Perhaps there is the sound of a ticking clock. [Pause.] Maybe you hear the class next door coming down the hall. [Pause.] Perhaps you hear a different sound. [Pause.] Try to notice what it is you are hearing."

For the super sense of seeing, let the children know that they may notice things that were always right there but they have never seen. Tell them, "We're going to begin by slowly letting your gaze travel around the room. Maybe you notice what color the walls are or where the heat comes from. Just slowly look around and really see what's in the room. Maybe you notice the clock and how it moves or what is on the wall near the windows or the shelves. Just slowly take it all in with your special power vision. And when we stop, let's close our eyes if that feels comfortable to you. Now, when I count to three, open them again and see how everything looks new and different!"

Then tell the children to get ready to explore their super-terrific touch—without even moving! Begin by saying, "If it feels all right, close your eyes. Take your attention to the temperature in our room and notice if it feels hot or cold. Maybe you can feel air

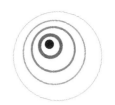

moving by and around you. [Pause.] Do you notice how the floor feels to you as you sit on it? Maybe you even can feel the bones in your bottom pressing against the floor. Let your attention move to your skin and notice the feel of your clothes on your skin. [Pause.] Perhaps they feel itchy, warm, or soft. We're just noticing what we don't usually notice and seeing how it feels."

Feel free to follow up with scent as well!

You can find other excellent guided meditations for children in the book *Spinning Inward: Using Guided Imagery with Children for Learning, Creativity & Relaxation* by Maureen Murdock (Shambhala 1987) and the CD *Yoga Child: A Peaceful Place Inside* (Bingo Kids 2006), available on Spotify. Two other good books to check out are *I Am Peace: A Book of Mindfulness* by Susan Verde (Abrams Books for Young Readers 2017) and *Peaceful Piggy Meditation* by Kerry Lee MacLean (Albert Whitman & Company 2004). You can also find helpful books, videos, and other materials at www.plumvillage.org.

ENHANCING SELF-REGULATION SKILLS

So far we've talked about yoga as a group activity. Another great way to use yoga is on an as-needed basis with children who need a moment to regain their self-regulation skills. Children often lash out because they feel emotions rising in their bodies. Yoga gives them a chance to separate the emotion from a possible negative reaction so they can respond in more appropriate ways. Whatever techniques you use for managing individual behaviors or handling conflict in your classroom, yoga can enhance children's ability to maintain their self-control.

If you see a child's emotions starting to get the best of him or her, you might be able to nip a problem in the bud by leading the child in a breath or a yoga pose. A well-timed "Elliott, give me three deep breaths" can be the difference that allows the child to

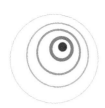

keep control over his behavior. Instructing him to put his hand on his belly while he breathes helps him focus his energy on calming down. If a few children are getting agitated during free play, interrupting to lead them all in a brief *Tree* pose is a light-hearted way to redirect their attention and energy. Do it along with them, with a grin.

Once children have lost their cool, they may need to be removed from a situation or activity. Suggest using yoga during this time to give them something positive to do that directly affects their emotions and behavior. Yoga has the potential to accelerate and deepen children's ability to regain their equilibrium. You can suggest a few simple deep breaths or a more involved activity. Review chapters 3 and 4 for calming suggestions. *Open-and-Shut Breath*, *Bird Breath*, and *Slurping Breath* are options. So are for-ward-bending poses such as *Rock*, *Gorilla*, and *Sea Star*. Children could do a quiet version of *Butterfly-Flutterby*, where the knees stay still and the back and head lean gently forward toward the feet. When a child is feeling too angry for a calming pose, a few *Dino Breaths* can be just the ticket to help him or her release the heat.

You can suggest yoga activities as the need arises or adopt one as your class's go-to so children know to begin that breath or pose whenever they are removed from the group due to behavior. Children might even start to do the pose or breath on their own, perhaps heading off the need to be removed from the group. Remember, yoga is an internal as well as physical activity. The purpose of these self-regulating activities is for children to feel better inside their bodies, as well as regain their place with their class.

CHAPTER 6

You Are You and I Am Me—Activities for Children of Differing Abilities

Once upon a time, this chapter would have been for teachers of children with "special needs." It does describe techniques that allow you to teach some yoga to most children, even if they have a disability. Research supports doing so, as yoga has been shown to be especially valuable for children with special needs (Mochan 2017). These days, however, virtually every preschool classroom includes children who are differently abled physically,

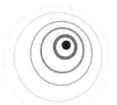

cognitively, emotionally, and/or behaviorally. Being familiar with techniques for doing yoga with these children is a valuable tool for everyone to have.

The last few decades have seen a dramatic upswing in children with various disorders. If you are a longtime teacher, you have likely witnessed this increase firsthand, and the numbers support your observations. The Centers for Disease Control (CDC) reports that as of 2016, one in every six children in the United States ages two to eight has a mental health issue, most commonly attention deficit hyperactivity disorder (ADHD), behavioral problems, anxiety, and depression (CDC 2019).

You may know that autism spectrum disorder (ASD) is also on the rise. In 2014 the CDC reported that by the age of eight, about one in every sixty-eight children in the United States had been identified with ASD. About half of those children received their diagnosis by the time they were four and a half. Even more, 80 percent, had documented developmental difficulties by the time they turned three. By comparison, in the years 2000–2002, the number of children identified with ASD was less than half the number identified in 2014, about one in every 150 eight-year-olds (Baio et al. 2018). At the same time, we educators are becoming much more knowledgeable about differences in brain development and the sometimes subtle ways in which children may have difficulty

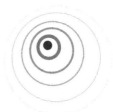

processing and acting on information. This means that behavioral and learning differences among preschoolers are now fairly common.

Many children in your class who experience these issues may not have a formal diagnosis, so it's up to you to notice what their behavior may be telling you. In some cases, a child who is seemingly not focused or who refuses to take part in an activity may be communicating that something about it is a challenge. For example, a child who demonstrates avoidance by refusing to participate may have unrecognized anxiety, especially if this child also shows separation struggles, frequent crying, refusal to talk at times (selective mutism), inflexibility, and moodiness. A child who acts out in a physical way may also be anxious or dealing with some trauma. Or it may be that a child won't try to do something out of fear of embarrassment or belief that he or she simply can't do it. (This is common with adults, too, for that matter.) Children who appear not to process information, or who respond in a very different way than expected, may be sending you the message that they have some form of differing ability. If some children struggle with poses more than others, it may be that you are seeing the results of low muscle tone, gross-motor planning difficulties, or weakness through the core muscle group. Some children may become overly excited during yoga and exhibit repetitive movement or "flapping." This may be a form of the restricted, repetitive behavior that is associated with ASD, especially when accompanied by social communication challenges.

Fortunately, yoga can help. As we've been discussing throughout this book, yoga promotes self-regulation, gross-motor skill and planning, vestibular and proprioceptive integration, self-discovery, physical and mental focus, strength and flexibility, self-esteem, and reduction of anxiety. (The vestibular system is the sensory system that provides the sense of balance and spatial orientation for the purpose of coordinating movement and balance. Proprioception is the ability to sense the positioning of body parts

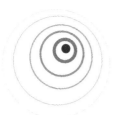

relative to one another and to our surroundings, as well as the strength of effort applied to movement. Pressure and force sometimes feel good because they are "giving information" to the body.) By promoting all of these skills, yoga benefits all children, including those with mental health disorders, cognitive challenges, and physical disabilities. All you need to do is teach it!

As teachers, we see the wholes of our children and what they *can* do rather than focusing on what they *cannot* do due to differing abilities. When we support them for success by recognizing the skills they have and helping them build on those skills for the future, we help these children create healthy feelings of connection and acceptance with their unique bodies. Yoga sets children up to recognize their own thoughts, create self-awareness, dissolve negative self-talk, and create a positive self-image. Even a child who uses a wheelchair or crutches or has other mobility challenges can be supported on a yoga journey.

This book does not go into depth about mental health disorders or other challenges children in your class may face, but the following overview gives some information on how yoga can be used to help support these children.

TEACHER TIME

Recognizing negative self-talk can be a powerful way to increase our own self-esteem. Try to stop every once in a while and notice the chatter going on in your head. Are you putting yourself down with self-negating comments like "I can't do this" or "I'm not as good as . . ."? Are you minimizing the work you do or the things you value? Or are you recognizing your good traits and the positive things you do? Do you ever tell yourself "I'm a great teacher" or "I am capable"? Negative self-talk is extremely common. Next time you find that the voice in your head is criticizing you, stop it and compliment yourself instead. Keep that up to develop the habit of being kinder to yourself.

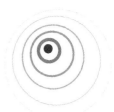

● **Children with, or who might have, ADHD.** Paying attention is an issue with these children, but they will usually have the required focus to be able to master poses (provided that you minimize major distractions). They likely find the deep breathing of yoga calming, and the movement allows the physical release they need in their bodies.

● **Children who exhibit behaviors associated with ASD.** Yoga can be especially beneficial for these children. It can reduce obsessive or repetitive behavior and can calm aggression and the need for self-stimulation, while at the same time helping with sensory integration (Brandstaetter 2014). Yoga supports communication because it uses visual prompts, and it promotes social interaction because it is a group activity in which each child occupies his or her own defined space.

● **Children who experience anxiety.** The self-regulation that comes from yoga poses, along with deep breathing, slows down the body's fight, flight, or freeze response, reducing symptoms. Yoga also causes children to focus in the moment; paying attention to matching his or her body to the pose you are doing can distract the child from worries.

● **Children who experience sensory processing or sensory-motor disorders.** Children's internal vestibular and proprioceptive systems are like compasses trying to keep them going in a specific direction. For children with these types of disorders, the compass is a bit off-kilter. Another way to think of this is as a cat without whiskers—children with these difficulties are missing pieces they need to make their way in the world with grace and coordination. Yoga helps reset the compass and replace some of the missing pieces. It allows the children's internal sensory systems to make better use of the information around them, moving them toward a state of equilibrium. Yogamagination can also help children with these types of learning difficulties.

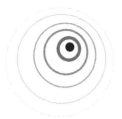

The movement brings sensory input that helps them pay attention to information in relevant ways, and they can learn concepts through the stories, such as sequencing and seeing the whole picture.

- **Children with postural disorder or dyspraxia.** These children are usually first identified due to poor motor planning, coordination, balance, and fine-motor skills, and difficulty crossing the midline. Yoga poses address all of these difficulties. These children will be aided by using their own body weight and developing core muscle strength.

- **Children who have cerebral palsy.** Yoga can strengthen the muscles of the limbs and the diaphragm, which supports deeper breathing and enables more movement for children with cerebral palsy. Yoga also benefits cognition and sensory processing, which can be affected by this disorder.

Children with the disorders described above are usually receptive to intervention strategies that bring movement and sound into play, which may have a calming effect. They also interpret input from muscles more easily than other forms of sensory input, such as hearing and seeing. Teaching these tools of movement integration and mindfulness in the early childhood classroom can set the foundation for self-regulation (Mochan 2017).

Children with autism, ADHD, or conduct disorders have difficulty with transitions. Often, yoga benefits classroom management by easing them into a transition, as mentioned in previous chapters.

AWARENESS TECHNIQUES

For the techniques described below, visual prompts are critical. They are a key tool that helps support children with differing abilities, whether you demonstrate the pose, show flash cards, or

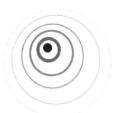

display pictures. When demonstrating an activity, it helps to go a little over the top so that there is no way the children can't hear or see exactly what you are doing!

Breathing and Poses to Increase Body Awareness and Spatial Relations

Breathing is simple and very important here. The number one thing to keep in mind is to demonstrate, letting your belly balloon and being audible so they hear you breathing.

The most helpful direction is to ask the children to breathe in and out with a hand on their bellies. This allows them to feel how their belly buttons push away from their backs when they breathe in, and how their belly buttons pull to their backbones when they breathe out. It gives anatomical awareness and helps develop the muscles of the core grouping, which ultimately supports the poses.

Poses that allow kids to bear their own weight increase body and spatial awareness with both proprioceptive and vestibular input. Balancing and weight-bearing poses are great for proprioceptive input, such as *Airplane*, *Downward Dog*, *Let's Fly a Kite*, *L on the Wall*, *Let It Rain*, *Stormy Weather*, *London Bridge*, *Mountain*, *Teapot*, *Tickle Toes*, *Tree*, *Warmth of the Sun*, *Warrior*, and *Yoga Roll-Ups*.

Moving, balancing, rocking, and jumping poses give vestibular input, such as *Gorilla Tapping*, *Hop to It*, *Horse*, *Let It Rain*, *Peaceful Piggy*, *Seashell*, *Row Your Boat*, *Satellite*, *Seesaw*, *Tickle Toes*, and *Wheels on the Bus*.

Be aware that you have the job of coregulation, and too much rolling, rocking, or bouncing can overstimulate vestibular information. Finding an energetic balance between the standing and balancing poses is where you can make the most of these poses for both proprioception and vestibular integration.

Breathing, Poses, and Activities to Stimulate the Sense of Touch

Touch is a touchy subject, and this is especially true for many children with differing abilities. Some are resistant to touching certain things, some may not be comfortable placing a whole foot on the ground, and some need pressure for their nervous systems to better process information. Their responses will be varied, but with poses, breath, and using your reassuring voice to guide the experience, touch can be soothing and also help children integrate sensory input.

Ocean Friends

Begin this very helpful breathing exercise by inviting the children to lie on their backs. With their permission, place bean bags on their bellies so they have something tangible to connect them to the rise and fall of their breathing. Invite them to feel the rise and fall of their bellies as they breathe.

Smooshy Ball

This well-received activity, best for small groups, is extremely helpful for sensory integration. It uses the light but firm pressure of a ball rolling down the children's spines. Invite the children onto their bellies. Tell them they are going to try something very special if they can let their bodies be still.

With a large ball, start at the top of the shoulders, and applying gentle pressure, roll the ball down each child's back slowly, hand over hand, avoiding pressure on the joints. Roll it back up and then down again. As with anything, always give children the choice to opt out of this activity. They may first need to watch and observe something new and different.

Yoga Roll-Ups

This small-group activity requires mats. If you have them, this is something your groups will probably ask for again and again.

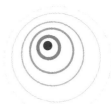

Invite the children to lie across the mat at one end. You and coteachers or assistants will roll them up in the mat, and after a moment, unroll them. So much fun, and learning with a purpose too!

PROMPTS AND CHOREOGRAPHING THE EXPERIENCE

When it comes to poses, most lend themselves to the sense of touch. It is just a matter of using your words as prompts to support the children's discovery of what they feel in a pose. Little bellies, feet, hands, and backs are all in contact with the ground at different points, and you can use your words to highlight these areas and bring the children's awareness to what they are feeling.

Using your words to set the stage for self-discovery during these and other poses and activities might sound like this:

"Press your feet down and spread your toes like tree roots in the soil."

"Spread your fingers on the ground like tiger paws."

"Push the sky with the top of your head."

"Reach high and tickle the sky."

"Lying on your belly, take a breath and feel your belly push the ground."

"When you rock and roll, feel your backbone touch the ground."

"Push your feet down into the ground."

"Pull your belly button back to your back."

"Push your belly out and feel it push your hand."

"What parts of your body can you feel touch the ground?"

"Can you feel the air move around you?"

You may be able to think of a few on your own!

SOUND, QUIET, AND THE INNER CONNECTION IN BREATHING POSES

The sound of the breath is something a baby hears as soon as the ears are developed enough to hear his or her own mother's breath in the womb. It is calming and familiar. Once young children make the connection to the action of their breath and can feel the expansion and contraction and hear the sound, they begin to recognize that they can use it to regulate their emotional climate, even at an early age. This is one of the best gifts we can give our children in their lifetimes. It will enable them to be happier, healthier, and more adaptable.

Any of the breathing techniques described in chapter 3 can be used. You can also invite children to take three mindful, aware breaths together. Counting "one, two, three" as they breathe out can bring them back into themselves and allow them to feel a shift in their energy. When they make the exhale audible by opening their mouths and releasing with a little sigh, you can see their shoulders drop, showing a release of tension. Even the youngest yoga students do this and enjoy the audible release of sound. Some verbal prompts may come in handy, such as asking the children if they can hear their breath or if they can notice that it sounds like waves at the beach.

Another important sound that can be used in poses is the sound of the voice. There is a deep connection between certain sounds and our own inner worlds. Adult yoga classes may use a mantra, also called seed syllables, that can affect the inner body. Sounds made by bells or singing bowls ring a certain pitch that resonates within the body. If you are skeptical about the power of sound, here are some stories to persuade you!

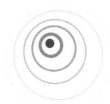

- A teacher frequently used chanting in a prenatal yoga class. When the moms brought their beautiful wee ones to visit and the infants heard the teacher's voice, those young children showed that they recognized the sound of the teacher's voice.

- In another situation, the same teacher was working with a six-year-old child who showed the significant motor and cognitive disability of Rett syndrome. He appeared unable to respond, always had a hand in his mouth, and was quite spastic in movement. The teacher placed the child's bare foot on her throat while humming different frequencies. It was possibly the only way to connect. The child moved his head, opened his eyes wide, and focused for the first time on the teacher! When she did this repeatedly, he would take his hands out of his mouth, and his uncontrolled movement slowed. Clearly the child felt a connection with this teacher, created through sound.

We talked earlier about breath and body awareness, then breath and touch. Now we turn to the sound of the breath, the most important sound when doing poses. Tell the children, "Let's take three yoga breaths in and out," just about every time you start a new pose. You can invite them to release the breath out of their mouths with an audible sound, like a sigh. Encourage them to recognize the sound of the exhale.

You also can use the vibration of the voice to help them recognize that sound can be felt within their bodies. Try chanting the alphabet in small increments. Inhale, place hands on heart or tummy, and then chant the sound of a letter throughout the exhale. When the breath is fully out, the sound stops. Then move on to the next letter. You can also use this chanting technique to buzz like a bee or hoot like an owl. Ask the children if they feel the letter sound inside. Ask them if the letters or sounds felt different from one another. You may also have the children

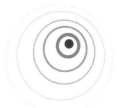

cover their ears with their palms and hum, and then have them take their hands off their ears and hum to notice the difference between the sounds.

Depending on the regulations of your setting, you might invite a child who is struggling to make a connection to put a hand on your throat and feel the vibration from your voice.

Using chimes or a singing bowl can be a lovely way for children to connect to sound. You may even ask the children to show you where they feel a sound by placing a hand on that part of their body, helping them connect awareness to vibration within the body.

Introducing yoga to these children can provide profound experiences for you and for your children. Making that breakthrough connection with a child who is severely disabled is one of the most poignant moments a yoga teacher could ever have.

Conclusion:
Yoga, Mindfulness,
and Self-Awareness

Yoga is, in reality, a science—the science of self-awareness. The ancient yogis knew this, and the information is here for us to teach to children in our classrooms and use ourselves. The scientific community is beginning to study and prove what the ancients knew—that learning to slow down our minds and bodies, bringing them toward stillness, can ultimately make us happier, healthier, and more well-adjusted individuals, whether we are four years old or forty. Yoga and mindfulness teach us to go inward, notice the sound of our breath, and ultimately still the chatter that the mind likes to feed us on a loop. It's never too early to begin this important skill. This mental chatter is what very often creates anxiety, stress, or anger, though often what it's telling us isn't real. The mind may create a whole narrative about something in the future that hasn't even happened yet, and if we buy into it instead of stepping away, we may become anxious. Or the mind may tell us a version of something that happened long ago—or yesterday—that makes us unhappy. It may or may not be true, but it's a form of negative self-talk. Children do it just like adults do.

Yoga techniques teach all of us, children and adults alike, that we can become aware of our bodies and the emotions and sensations we feel in them by making a connection to our breath and moving toward stillness. Then we can start to know how we want to respond to our surroundings in ways that will benefit us and those around us. Reaching that point allows us to find the freedom that comes from being present for ourselves and others, and enjoy the peace that comes from connecting to the people and world around us. We see it in our students when they learn to calm themselves after an altercation with a classmate, talk it out, smile, and go on playing. We can see it in ourselves when we let go of small resentments and anxieties and allow room for more joy in our lives. Pretty wonderful, right?

If you have reached this page, you have probably come to your own conclusions about how the material in this book is going to benefit your young learners and yourself. Maybe you already go to yoga classes and know just how great you feel after. Or perhaps you are at a point where you are seeking ways to support emotional growth and self-regulation for your students. Maybe you are just curious because you have heard a lot about the words *yoga* or *mindfulness*. This book provides the ideas, format, poses, and functions for how you might bring yoga and mindfulness into your classroom to share with your children and perhaps even their families as well. Whatever your reason for reading this book, the time is ripe to create change, and it can start with you.

That said, please don't overthink starting your yoga program or allow your inner critic to tell you that you aren't capable of bringing these concepts into your day-to-day classroom life. Even if you do not practice yoga currently, you can do this. It does not matter if you are flexible physically. Remember, Rome wasn't built in a day, and neither is a new program or way of doing things. The key is to start small; small changes support big growth over time. Begin simply by making changes that will shift your classroom toward a kinder, more conscious place where your children's physical, social, and emotional learning is enhanced. Everyone will be happier for it.

Start by implementing just one or two techniques. No, there won't be an immediate transformation, but you will see change. Allow yourself to get comfortable with the activities you choose, and then when you feel comfortable, add two more. Build slow and grow, grow, grow. This book is the seed that, carefully tended, will sprout into something beautiful.

Recommended Resources

If you are interested in learning more about yoga for adults or young children, these books and websites are great places to start.

Comprehensive Yoga Therapy: Attending to Your Whole Self by Ilene S. Rosen, Robert Butera, and Jennifer Hilbert (Woodbury, MN: Llewellyn Publications, 2020).

I Am Peace: A Book of Mindfulness by Susan Verde (New York: Abrams Books for Young Readers, 2017).

Mindful Bea and the Worry Tree by Gail Silver (Washington, DC: Magination Press, 2019).

Peaceful Piggy Meditation by Kerry Lee MacLean (Park Ridge, IL: Albert Whitman & Company, 2004).

The Pure Heart of Yoga: Ten Essential Steps for Personal Transformation by Robert Butera (Woodbury, MN: Llewellyn Publications, 2009).

Spinning Inward: Using Guided Imagery with Children for Learning, Creativity & Relaxation by Maureen Murdock (Boulder, CO: Shambhala, 1987).

Steps and Stones: An Anh's Anger Story by Gail Silver (Berkeley, CA: Plum Blossom Books, 2007).

Yoga and Mindfulness for Young Children, a website featuring tools and tips from this book's authors. http://www.mothergoose andthemadhatter.net.

Yoga Child: A Peaceful Place Inside (Bingo Kids, 2006).

Yoga for Dummies by Larry Payne and Georg Feuerstein (Hoboken, NJ: John Wiley & Sons, 2014).

The Yoga-Sūtra of Patañjali: A New Translation and Commentary (Rochester, VT: Inner Traditions, 1989).

Yoga Therapy for Stress and Anxiety by Robert Butera, Erin Byron, and Staffan Elgelid (Woodbury, MN: Llewellyn Publications, 2015).

You can also find helpful books, videos, and other materials at www.plumvillage.org.

Index of Poses

Name	Position	Primary Attribute	Page #
Breathing Activities			
Belly Breath		Calm, Refocus	29
Bird Breath		Calm, Lung Expansion	31
Bunny Breath		Energize	33
Buzzing Breath		Release Anger, Fun	33
Catch a Ball Breath		Energize	34
Dino Breath		Release Anger	34
Open-and-Shut Breath		Calm, Uplift	31
Slurping Breath		Calm, Cool	32
Snakey Breath		Cool, Calm, Fun	32
Wave Breath		Calm or Energize	34
Brain Breaks			
Half Star to Star			77
Reach the Sky			77
Stop, Drop, and Rock			78
Twinkle, Little Star			78
Wiggly Worm			78
Yoga Fun and Games			
The Bell Game			79
Clear the Clouds			79
Going on a Bear Hunt			80
Head, Shoulders, Knees, and Toes			81
Monkey See, Monkey Do			82
Monkey Toes			82
Skidamarinky Dinky Dink, Skidamarinky Do			83
We're All Connected			83
Yoga Bear Says			84

Name	Position	Primary Attribute	Page #
Yogamaginations, Gross Motor			
Balance			88
Body Awareness/Proprioception			89
Calming 1 and 2			89–90
Energy 1 and 2			90–91
Gross Motor 1 and 2			91–92
Strength 1 and 2			92–93
Yogamaginations, Curriculum			
Down on the Farm			97
I Like Me			98
Let's All Come Together			99
The Rain Forest 1 and 2			100–101
Spring Walk			95
Transformation Station			101
Trip to the Zoo			102
Yogamaginations, Act Out a Story			
Guided Imagery			
Happy Heart			108
I Can Do Anything			110
Magic Carpet			108
Monkey Toes			82
Ocean			107
Peaceful Paws			110
The Rainbow			111
Skidamarinky Dinky Dink, Skidamarinky Do			83
Superspecial Senses			111
We're All Connected			83
Yoga Bear Says			84

References

Baio, Jon, et al. 2018. "Prevalence of Autism Spectrum Disorder among Children Aged 8 Years—Autism and Developmental Disabilities Monitoring Network, 11 Sites, United States, 2014." *Morbidity and Mortality Weekly Report* 67 (6): 1–23. Centers for Disease Control and Prevention. www.cdc.gov/mmwr /volumes/67/ss/ss6706a1.htm.

Brandstaetter, Hannah. 2014. "Yoga Generates Huge Benefits for Children with Autism." *Yoga International*, October 30.

Centers for Disease Control and Prevention. 2019. "Data and Statistics on Children's Mental Health." Last reviewed April 19, 2019. www.cdc.gov/childrensmentalhealth/data.html.

Mochan, Michelle. 2017. "The Benefits of Teaching Yoga to Young Children with Special Needs: Developing an Appropriate Methodology." *International Journal of Technology and Inclusive Education (IJTIE)* 6 (2): 1161–70.

Patañjali. 1989. *The Yoga-Sūtra of Patañjali: A New Translation and Commentary.* Translated by Georg Feuerstein. Rochester, VT: Inner Traditions, Bear and Company.

Razza, Rachel A., Dessa K. Bergen-Cico, and Kimberly Raymond. 2015. "Enhancing Preschoolers' Self-Regulation via Mindful Yoga." *Journal of Child and Family Studies* 24 (2): 372–85. https://doi.org/10.1007/s10826-013-9847-6.

Shonkoff, Jack P., Andrew S. Garner, and the Committee on Psychosocial Aspects of Child and Family Health, Committee on Early Childhood, Adoption, and Dependent Care, and Section on Developmental and Behavioral Pediatrics, Benjamin S. Siegel, Mary I. Dobbins, Marian F. Earls, Laura McGuinn, John Pascoe, and David L. Wood. 2012. "The Lifelong Effects of Early Childhood Adversity and Toxic Stress." *Pediatrics* 129 (1): e232–e246. http://pediatrics.aappublications.org/content/129/1/e232.